T0226968

Disease Prevention

Editors

MICHAEL P. PIGNONE
KIRSTEN BIBBINS-DOMINGO

MEDICAL CLINICS
OF NORTH AMERICA

www.medical.theclinics.com

Consulting Editor
BIMAL H. ASHAR

July 2017 • Volume 101 • Number 4

ELSEVIER

1600 John F. Kennedy Boulevard ● Suite 1800 ● Philadelphia, Pennsylvania, 19103-2899

http://www.theclinics.com

MEDICAL CLINICS OF NORTH AMERICA Volume 101, Number 4
July 2017 ISSN 0025-7125, ISBN-13: 978-0-323-53138-2

Editor: Jessica McCool
Developmental Editor: Alison Swety

Medical Clinics of North America (ISSN 0025-7125) is published bimonthly by Elsevier Inc., 360 Park Avenue South, New York, NY 10010-1710. Months of publication are January, March, May, July, September, and November. Business and editorial offices: 1600 John F. Kennedy Boulevard, Suite 1800, Philadelphia, PA 19103-2899. Periodicals postage paid at New York, NY, and additional mailing offices. Subscription prices are USD $268.00 per year (US individuals), $563.00 per year (US institutions), $100.00 per year (US Students), $330.00 per year (Canadian individuals), $731.00 per year (Canadian institutions), $200.00 per year (Canadian and foreign students), $402.00 per year (foreign individuals), and $731.00 per year (foreign institutions). To receive student/resident rate, orders must be accompanied by name of affiliated institution, date of term, and the signature of program/residency coordinator on institution letterhead. Orders will be billed at individual rate until proof of status is received. Foreign air speed delivery is included in all Clinics' subscription prices. All prices are subject to change without notice. **POSTMASTER:** Send address changes to *Medical Clinics of North America*, Elsevier Health Sciences Division, Subscription Customer Service, 3251 Riverport Lane, Maryland Heights, MO 63043. **Customer Service: Telephone: 1-800-654-2452** (U.S. and Canada); **1-314-447-8871** (outside U.S. and Canada). **Fax: 314-447-8029. E-mail: journalscustomerserviceusa@elsevier.com** (for print support); **journalsonlinesupport-usa@elsevier.com** (for online support).

Reprints. For copies of 100 or more of articles in this publication, please contact the Commercial Reprints Department, Elsevier Inc., 360 Park Avenue South, New York, NY 10010-1710. Tel.: 212-633-3874; Fax: 212-633-3820; E-mail: reprints@elsevier.com.

Medical Clinics of North America is also published in Spanish by McGraw-Hill Interamericana Editores S. A., P.O. Box 5-237, 06500 Mexico, D.F., Mexico.

Medical Clinics of North America is covered in *MEDLINE/PubMed (Index Medicus), Current Contents, ASCA, Excerpta Medica, Science Citation Index,* and *ISI/BIOMED.*

PROGRAM OBJECTIVE
The goal of the *Medical Clinics of North America* is to keep practicing physicians up to date with current clinical practice by providing timely articles reviewing the state of the art in patient care.

TARGET AUDIENCE
All practicing physicians and other healthcare professionals.

LEARNING OBJECTIVES
Upon completion of this activity, participants will be able to:
1. Review recommendations for prevention of cardiovascular disease.
2. Discuss screening for lung, cervical, and colorectal cancers, among others.
3. Recognize methods for screening for depression, unhealthy alcohol use, and other diseases.

ACCREDITATION
The Elsevier Office of Continuing Medical Education (EOCME) is accredited by the Accreditation Council for Continuing Medical Education (ACCME) to provide continuing medical education for physicians.

The EOCME designates this enduring material for a maximum of 15 *AMA PRA Category 1 Credit*(s)™. Physicians should claim only the credit commensurate with the extent of their participation in the activity.

All other healthcare professionals requesting continuing education credit for this enduring material will be issued a certificate of participation.

DISCLOSURE OF CONFLICTS OF INTEREST
The EOCME assesses conflict of interest with its instructors, faculty, planners, and other individuals who are in a position to control the content of CME activities. All relevant conflicts of interest that are identified are thoroughly vetted by EOCME for fair balance, scientific objectivity, and patient care recommendations. EOCME is committed to providing its learners with CME activities that promote improvements or quality in healthcare and not a specific proprietary business or a commercial interest.

The planning committee, staff, authors and editors listed below have identified no financial relationships or relationships to products or devices they or their spouse/life partner have with commercial interest related to the content of this CME activity:
Kirsten Bibbins-Domingo, PhD, MD, MAS; Alison T. Brenner, PhD, MPH; Linda E. Chen, MD; Michael Dougherty, MD; Anjali Fortna; James C. Garbutt, MD; Richard M. Hoffman, MD, MPH; Megan J. Huchko, MD, MPH; Daniel E. Jonas, MD, MPH; Dhruv S. Kazi, MD, MSc, MS; Christoph I. Lee, MD, MS; Jessica McCool; Andrew E. Moran, MD, MPH; Douglas K. Owens, MD, MS; Joanne M. Penko, MS, MPH; Michael P. Pignone, MD, MPH; Mark J. Pletcher, MD, MPH; Daniel S. Reuland, MD, MPH; Ilana B. Richman, MD; Rolando Sanchez, MD; George F. Sawaya, MD; Leigh H. Simmons, MD; Sarah Smithson, MD, MPH; Jeyanthi Surendrakumar; Alison Swety; Anthony J. Viera, MD, MPH; Katie Widmeier; Amy Williams.

The planning committee, staff, authors and editors listed below have identified financial relationships or relationships to products or devices they or their spouse/life partner have with commercial interest related to the content of this CME activity:
Michael J. Barry, MD, MACP has research support from, and an employment affiliation with, Healthwise, Incorporated, and is a consultant/advisor for Risk Management Foundation and the National Cancer Institute at the National Institutes of Health.
Joann G. Elmore, MD, MPH receives royalties/patents from Wolters Kluwer.

UNAPPROVED/OFF-LABEL USE DISCLOSURE
The EOCME requires CME faculty to disclose to the participants:
1. When products or procedures being discussed are off-label, unlabelled, experimental, and/or investigational (not US Food and Drug Administration [FDA] approved); and
2. Any limitations on the information presented, such as data that are preliminary or that represent ongoing research, interim analyses, and/or unsupported opinions. Faculty may discuss information about pharmaceutical agents that is outside of FDA-approved labelling. This information is intended solely for CME and is not intended to promote off-label use of these medications. If you have any questions, contact the medical affairs department of the manufacturer for the most recent prescribing information.

TO ENROLL
To enroll in the *Medical Clinics of North America* Continuing Medical Education program, call customer service at 1-800-654-2452 or sign up online at http://www.theclinics.com/home/cme. The CME program is available to subscribers for an additional annual fee of USD $295.

METHOD OF PARTICIPATION

In order to claim credit, participants must complete the following:

1. Complete enrolment as indicated above.
2. Read the activity.
3. Complete the CME Test and Evaluation. Participants must achieve a score of 70% on the test. All CME Tests and Evaluations must be completed online.

CME INQUIRIES/SPECIAL NEEDS

For all CME inquiries or special needs, please contact elsevierCME@elsevier.com.

MEDICAL CLINICS OF NORTH AMERICA

RELATED INTEREST

Infectious Disease Clinics, September 2016 (Vol. 30, Issue 3)
**Infection Prevention and Control in Healthcare,
Part I: Facility Planning and Management**
Keith S. Kaye and Sorabh Dhar, *Editors*
Available at: http://www.id.theclinics.com/

Infectious Disease Clinics, December 2016 (Vol. 30, Issue 4)
**Infection Prevention and Control in Healthcare,
Part II: Epidemiology and Prevention of Infections**
Keith S. Kaye and Sorabh Dhar, *Editors*
Available at: http://www.id.theclinics.com/

THE CLINICS ARE AVAILABLE ONLINE!
Access your subscription at:
www.theclinics.com

Contributors

CONSULTING EDITOR

BIMAL H. ASHAR, MD, MBA, FACP
Associate Professor of Medicine, Division of General Internal Medicine, Johns Hopkins University School of Medicine, Baltimore, Maryland

EDITORS

MICHAEL P. PIGNONE, MD, MPH
Professor of Medicine and Chair, Department of Internal Medicine, Dell Medical School, The University of Texas at Austin, Austin, Texas

KIRSTEN BIBBINS-DOMINGO, PhD, MD, MAS
Lee Goldman, MD Endowed Chair in Medicine, Professor of Medicine, Departments of Medicine, and Epidemiology and Biostatistics, University of California, San Francisco, UCSF Center for Vulnerable Populations, Division of General Internal Medicine, Zuckerberg San Francisco General Hospital, San Francisco, California

AUTHORS

MICHAEL J. BARRY, MD, MACP
Professor of Medicine, Part-time, Harvard Medical School, General Medicine Division, Massachusetts General Hospital, Boston, Massachusetts

KIRSTEN BIBBINS-DOMINGO, PhD, MD, MAS
Lee Goldman, MD Endowed Chair in Medicine, Professor of Medicine, Departments of Medicine, and Epidemiology and Biostatistics, University of California, San Francisco, UCSF Center for Vulnerable Populations, Division of General Internal Medicine, Zuckerberg San Francisco General Hospital, San Francisco, California

ALISON T. BRENNER, PhD, MPH
Research Scientist, Cecil G Sheps Center for Health Services Research, Lineberger Comprehensive Cancer Center, University of North Carolina, Chapel Hill, North Carolina

LINDA E. CHEN, MD
Resident, Department of Radiology, University of Washington School of Medicine, Seattle, Washington

MICHAEL DOUGHERTY, MD
Fellow, Division of Gastroenterology and Hepatology, Department of Medicine, University of North Carolina, Chapel Hill, North Carolina

JOANN G. ELMORE, MD, MPH
Professor, Department of Medicine, University of Washington School of Medicine, Department of Epidemiology, University of Washington School of Public Health, Seattle, Washington

JAMES C. GARBUTT, MD
Professor, Department of Psychiatry, UNC Bowles Center for Alcohol Studies, School of Medicine, University of North Carolina, Chapel Hill, Chapel Hill, North Carolina

RICHARD M. HOFFMAN, MD, MPH
Professor, Department of Medicine, University of Iowa Carver College of Medicine, Holden Comprehensive Cancer Center, Iowa City, Iowa

MEGAN J. HUCHKO, MD, MPH
Associate Professor, Department of Obstetrics and Gynecology, Global Health Institute, Duke University, Durham, North Carolina

DANIEL E. JONAS, MD, MPH
Associate Professor, Department of Medicine, Director, Program on Medical Practice and Prevention, Cecil G. Sheps Center for Health Services Research, University of North Carolina, Chapel Hill, Chapel Hill, North Carolina

DHRUV S. KAZI, MD, MSc, MS
Associate Professor, Departments of Medicine, and Epidemiology and Biostatistics, University of California, San Francisco, UCSF Center for Vulnerable Populations, UCSF Center for Healthcare Value, Division of Cardiology, Zuckerberg San Francisco General Hospital, San Francisco, California

CHRISTOPH I. LEE, MD, MS
Associate Professor, Departments of Medicine, and Epidemiology and Biostatistics, University of California, San Francisco, UCSF Center for Vulnerable Populations, UCSF Center for Healthcare Value, Division of Cardiology, Zuckerberg San Francisco General Hospital, San Francisco, California

ANDREW E. MORAN, MD, MPH
Assistant Professor of Medicine, Division of General Medicine, Columbia University Medical Center, New York, New York

DOUGLAS K. OWENS, MD, MS
VA Palo Alto Health Care System, Palo Alto, California; Henry J. Kaiser, Junior Professor, Department of Medicine, Stanford University School of Medicine, Center for Primary Care and Outcomes Research/Center for Health Policy, Stanford, California

JOANNE M. PENKO, MS, MPH
Senior Research Analyst, UCSF Center for Vulnerable Populations, University of California, San Francisco, Division of General Internal Medicine, Zuckerberg San Francisco General Hospital, San Francisco, California

MICHAEL P. PIGNONE, MD, MPH
Professor of Medicine and Chair, Department of Internal Medicine, Dell Medical School, The University of Texas at Austin, Austin, Texas

MARK J. PLETCHER, MD, MPH
Professor of Epidemiology & Biostatistics and Medicine, University of California, San Francisco, San Francisco, California

DANIEL S. REULAND, MD, MPH
Professor of Medicine, Division of Internal Medicine and Clinical Epidemiology, Department of Medicine, Lineberger Comprehensive Cancer Center, University of North Carolina, Chapel Hill, North Carolina

ILANA B. RICHMAN, MD
Instructor, Department of Medicine, Yale University School of Medicine, New Haven, Connecticut

ROLANDO SANCHEZ, MD
Clinical Assistant Professor, Department of Medicine, University of Iowa Carver College of Medicine, Iowa City, Iowa

GEORGE F. SAWAYA, MD
Professor, Department of Obstetrics, Gynecology and Reproductive Sciences, Epidemiology & Biostatistics, University of California, San Francisco, San Francisco, California

LEIGH H. SIMMONS, MD
Assistant Professor of Medicine, Harvard Medical School, General Medicine Division, Massachusetts General Hospital, Boston, Massachusetts

SARAH SMITHSON, MD, MPH
Assistant Professor, Department of Medicine, University of North Carolina, Chapel Hill, Chapel Hill, North Carolina

ANTHONY J. VIERA, MD, MPH
Professor, Department of Family Medicine, University of North Carolina, Chapel Hill, Chapel Hill, North Carolina

Contents

Cardiovascular risk assessment is fundamental to prevention of cardiovascular disease, because it helps determine the size of the potential benefits that might accrue to individual patients from use of statins, aspirin, and other preventive interventions. Current guidelines recommend specific algorithms for cardiovascular risk assessment that combine information from traditional risk factors including blood pressure, lipids, and smoking, along with age and sex and other factors. These algorithms are the subject of active research and controversy. This article addresses the rationale, current guidelines and use, and potential future directions of cardiovascular risk assessment.

Numerous large randomized clinical trials have shown that statin therapy is effective and safe for primary prevention of atherosclerotic cardiovascular disease (CVD) for adults aged 40 to 75 years and support the use of 10-year CVD risk as a means to identify individuals for treatment. Uncertainty exists in those older than 75 years who may be more likely to benefit because of their underlying CVD risk, but also face uncertain harms. Several high-quality mathematical simulation models have shown that statin therapy is cost-effective for primary prevention of atherosclerotic CVD. Despite effectiveness and safety, statins are underutilized for primary prevention.

Hypertension affects 1 in 3 American adults. Blood pressure (BP)-lowering therapy reduces the risk of cardiovascular disease. The United States Preventive Services Task Force recommends all adults be screened for hypertension. Most patients whose office BP is elevated should have out-of-office monitoring to confirm the diagnosis. Ambulatory BP monitoring is preferred for out-of-office measurement, but home BP monitoring is a reasonable alternative. Guidelines for treatment are stratified by age (<60 vs >60 years) and include cutoffs for recommended treatment BPs and target BP goals. Quality of hypertension care is improved by incorporating population health management using registries and medication titration.

Aspirin reduces the risk of nonfatal myocardial infarction and stroke, and the risk of colorectal cancer. Aspirin increases the risk of gastrointestinal and intracranial bleeding. The best available evidence supports initiating aspirin in select populations. In 2016, the US Preventive Services Task Force recommended initiating aspirin for the primary prevention of both cardiovascular disease and colorectal cancer among adults ages 50 to 59 who are at increased risk for cardiovascular disease. Adults 60 to 69 who are at increased cardiovascular disease risk may also benefit. There remains considerable uncertainty about whether younger and older patients may benefit.

The approach to breast cancer screening has changed over time from a general approach to a more personalized, risk-based approach. Women with dense breasts, one of the most prevalent risk factors, are now being informed that they are at increased risk of developing breast cancer and should consider supplemental screening beyond mammography. This article reviews the current evidence regarding the impact of breast density relative to other known risk factors, the evidence regarding supplemental screening for women with dense breasts, supplemental screening options, and recommendations for physicians having shared decision-making discussions with women who have dense breasts.

Cervical cancer screening in the United States has accompanied profound decreases in cancer incidence and mortality over the last half century. Two screening strategies are currently endorsed by US-based guideline groups: (1) triennial cytology for women aged 21 to 65 years, and (2) triennial cytology for women aged 21 to 29 years followed by cytology plus testing for high-risk human papillomavirus types every 5 years for women aged 30 years and older. Providing women with affordable, easily accessible screening, follow-up of abnormal tests, and timely treatment will result in the greatest impact of screening on cervical cancer incidence and mortality.

Colorectal cancer (CRC) contributes a major burden of cancer mortality in the United States. There are multiple effective screening approaches that can reduce CRC mortality. These approaches are supported by different levels of evidence, and each has its own advantages and disadvantages.

Implementing a systematic approach to screening that addresses the multiple steps involved in the screening process is essential to improving population-level CRC screening. Offering patients stool-based screening is important for increasing screening uptake. However, programs that offer stool testing must support the population health infrastructure needed to promote adherence to repeat testing and follow-up of abnormal tests.

for health care providers. Well-validated screening instruments are available, and behavioral counseling interventions delivered in primary care can reduce risky drinking. For people with alcohol use disorder, treatment programs with or without medication can reduce consumption and promote abstinence. To overcome barriers to implementation of screening for alcohol use and subsequent delivery of appropriate interventions in primary care settings, support systems, changes in staffing or roles, formal protocols, and additional provider and staff training may be required.

Foreword

An Ounce of Prevention?

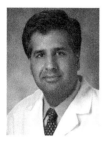

Bimal H. Ashar, MD, MBA, FACP
Consulting Editor

In the February 4, 1735 issue of the *Pennsylvania Gazette*, Benjamin Franklin wrote that "an ounce of prevention is worth a pound of cure." Mr Franklin was not referring to medicine when he penned the now-famous line. He instead was referring to the importance of fire safety and the need for the city of Philadelphia to be better prepared to prevent and react to fires. In his article, he noted the importance of tending to how hot coals were being transferred in shovels (primary prevention), how chimneys should be cleaned regularly (primary prevention), and how a "club or society of active men" (firefighters) should be formed who can efficiently extinguish fires (tertiary prevention).

Despite the original context of Mr Franklin's quotation, it has been used repeatedly in the field of medicine to stress the importance of disease prevention and early detection. The fundamental notion that preventing disease before it strikes holds significant value to patients and providers. Yet, primary prevention is often difficult and may require substantial lifestyle changes that challenge even the most devout patients. Early detection (secondary prevention) is even more controversial. If a disease is diagnosed in a presymptomatic phase, it would make sense that a better outcome would ensue. However, large trials have challenged this assumption. Concepts of lead time, length time, and overdiagnosis bias have emerged to explain the limited evidence for specific screening tests. Furthermore, if outcome is not improved, unnecessary harm may ensue due to morbidity and mortality from treatments that were not going to affect overall disease survival. Perhaps an ounce of prevention is not so valuable.

In this issue of *Medical Clinics of North America*, Drs Pignone and Bibbins-Domingo have enlisted an impressive group of experts to critically evaluate the preventive medicine literature. Emphasis has been placed on primary prevention of cardiovascular disease and cancer. However, the importance of other conditions seen in primary care practice has not been overlooked. Drs Jonas and Garbutt discuss the importance of

Med Clin N Am 101 (2017) xv–xvi
http://dx.doi.org/10.1016/j.mcna.2017.04.002
0025-7125/17/© 2017 Published by Elsevier Inc.

medical.theclinics.com

alcohol abuse screening, while Drs Smithson and Pignone elaborate on the utility of screening for depression. I am confident that this issue will serve as a valuable resource.

Bimal H. Ashar, MD, MBA, FACP
Division of General Internal Medicine
Johns Hopkins University School of Medicine
601 North Caroline Street
#7143
Baltimore, MD 21287, USA

E-mail address:
Bashar1@jhmi.edu

Preface

Update on Key Clinical Preventive Services for Adults

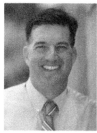
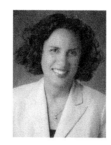

Michael P. Pignone, MD, MPH   Kirsten Bibbins-Domingo, PhD, MD, MAS
Editors

In this issue of *Medical Clinics of North America*, we present a series of articles on key issues in clinical preventive care for adults. The articles focus on primary prevention, with a mixture of screening, counseling, and use of preventive medications. We selected topics that are commonly encountered in clinical practice in the United States (and other developed countries), have substantial burdens of illness, and have robust evidence bases that allow assessment of the benefits and harms of potential interventions. We have focused this issue on three main topical areas: cardiovascular disease (CVD), cancer, and mental health.

In each article, the authors provide an assessment of the burden of disease for the target condition, data on the means of identifying the condition (where relevant), and a comprehensive assessment of the benefits and harms of potential interventions, including whether the evidence differs for different populations (eg, men vs women; different ages; or different risk levels). They review recommendations from major guideline-issuing organizations and provide guidance on how to most effectively implement recommendations in clinical practice.

Although each of the articles necessarily focuses on a single topic, primary care providers also need guidance on how to consider and implement an entire suite of preventive services in practice. Such a task is difficult in itself, more so when one considers that prevention is usually delivered along with acute illness care and the care of (often multiple) chronic conditions. It is no wonder that several studies have documented relatively low rates of delivery of evidence-based preventive services and the large time requirement for implementing all of the US Preventive (not Preventative) Services Task Force (USPSTF) recommended services within traditional organizational and financing structures.[1]

Fortunately, new research, new tools, and new methods for organizing and financing preventive care have become available to make delivering preventive care more

Med Clin N Am 101 (2017) xvii–xix
http://dx.doi.org/10.1016/j.mcna.2017.04.001
0025-7125/17/© 2017 Published by Elsevier Inc.   medical.theclinics.com

effective and efficient. This progress is well demonstrated in several of our topical areas. For example, in heart disease prevention, there is increasing acceptance that an approach to identification and management should rely on an assessment of overall (or "global") cardiovascular risk. Pletcher and Moran discuss the rationale for a risk-based approach to CVD prevention, note the availability of evidence-based risk calculators, and describe a novel method for deciding if a risk assessment based on traditional risk factors is sufficient, or whether novel risk markers should be added. Richman and Owens, in their review of aspirin for primary prevention, discuss how CVD risk and age can be used to help balance the benefits and harms of aspirin therapy; Kazi and colleagues examine a similar approach for the use of statins for primary prevention. Finally, Viera discusses the intricacies of how to use CVD risk to help guide treatment of hypertension, including how best to determine the threshold of blood pressure that warrants a recommendation for treatment or a recommendation for shared decision-making. However, each of the articles essentially considers its topic in isolation. The task of integrating and implementing the different CVD prevention recommendations, including the assessment of risk, in practice remains a challenge.

Recently, Maciosek and colleagues published helpful guidance for such integration and demonstrated how modeling can be used effectively to help providers understand the relative potential effects of different services.[2] They provide an assessment of the highest yield clinical preventive services, drawing from the list of USPSTF-recommended services (those receiving an "A" or "B" level recommendation). Their assessment was based on a combination of preventable burden of disease and judgment of the cost-effectiveness of potential interventions.

Not surprisingly, all four potential CVD prevention interventions for adults appeared among the top ten rankings: smoking cessation for adults (tied for first), aspirin prophylaxis (tied for fourth), and cholesterol and hypertension screening (tied for eighth), suggesting that primary care practices with large proportions of adult patients should focus efforts on the suite of CVD prevention services. Other topics covered in this issue also scored highly, including screening for alcohol misuse and screening for colorectal cancer. Notably, smoking cessation, tobacco use screening, alcohol misuse screening, and aspirin prophylaxis were all found to be cost-saving: that is, use of the service was associated with lower total costs than not implementing the service. Other highly rated services had cost-effectiveness ratios of $50,000 per quality-adjusted life-years (QALY) gained or better.

Maciosek and colleagues[2] also examined the number of potential QALYs that could be saved for a birth cohort of 4 million US adults if the service was implemented optimally (90% performance) rather than at its current level. They found that counseling to reduce tobacco use had the highest potential gain, followed by several of the preventive services reviewed in this issue: screening and counseling for alcohol misuse (140,000 QALYs), screening for colorectal cancer (110,000 QALYs), breast cancer screening (42,000 QALYs), aspirin prophylaxis (30,000 QALYs), and cervical cancer screening (14,000 QALYs). Current levels of screening for depression in adults were unclear, but conservatively estimating current performance at 50%, they found that optimal implementation could save 45,000 QALYs per birth cohort. These findings suggest there is great room for improvement in health through better implementation of clinical preventive services.

It is important to recognize that the costs of achieving optimal implementation have not been included in the cost-effectiveness models. The authors of the articles in this issue have noted some promising strategies for increasing appropriate use (and decreasing inappropriate use) of preventive services. The Centers for Disease Control and Prevention Guide to Community Preventive Services also provides excellent guidance for those wishing to increase the provision of high-value preventive services (www.communityguide.org). Techniques with strong evidence bases include use of audit and feedback (measuring and reporting back to providers their performance), clinical reminders directed to providers or to patients, use of small media, and reorganization of practice workflows. Financial incentives, directed to either providers or patients, have a mixed evidence base. More research is needed to better understand how different interventions may be combined most effectively and efficiently.

Michael P. Pignone, MD, MPH
Dell Medical School
The University of Texas at Austin
1912 Speedway
Mail Code D2000
Austin, TX 78712, USA

Kirsten Bibbins-Domingo, PhD, MD, MAS
University of California, San Francisco
Box 1364
San Francisco, CA 94143, USA

E-mail addresses:
pignone@austin.utexas.edu (M.P. Pignone)
kirsten.bibbins-domingo@ucsf.edu (K. Bibbins-Domingo)

REFERENCES

1. Yarnall KS, Pollak KI, Østbye T, et al. Primary care: is there enough time for prevention? Am J Public Health 2003;93(4):635–41.
2. Maciosek MV, LaFrance AB, Dehmer SP, et al. Updated priorities among effective clinical preventive services. Ann Fam Med 2017;15:14–22.

Cardiovascular Risk Assessment

Mark J. Pletcher, MD, MPH[a],*, Andrew E. Moran, MD, MPH[b]

KEYWORDS

- Cardiovascular risk • Risk prediction • Risk factors • Biomarkers
- Cardiovascular disease prevention

KEY POINTS

- Cardiovascular risk assessment can help guide targeted use of statins, aspirin, and other interventions to prevent cardiovascular disease.
- Risk equations that combine information from multiple cardiovascular risk factors can help clinicians estimate cardiovascular risk.
- The 2013 American College of Cardiology/American Heart Association Pooled Cohorts Risk Equations are the current standard in cardiovascular risk assessment, although they have been criticized for imperfect calibration.
- Novel risk factors, such as coronary artery calcium and C-reactive protein levels, can be used to further inform risk-based decision making.
- Clinicians should keep abreast of changes in recommendations for how and when to assess cardiovascular risk, because this is an active area of research.

INTRODUCTION

Cardiovascular risk assessment is fundamental to prevention of cardiovascular disease (CVD), the leading cause of morbidity and mortality in the United States.[1] Although some CVD prevention strategies are nearly universally beneficial and generally recommended (eg, healthy dietary and exercise habits, and smoking cessation among smokers),[2] others are associated with significant cost and/or potential risks for adverse effects (eg, preventive medications such as aspirin, antihypertensive medications, and statins), and are generally reserved for use in persons for whom the

Disclosure: Neither author has any relationship with a commercial company that has a direct financial interest in subject matter or materials discussed in article or with a company making a competing product.
[a] Departments of Epidemiology & Biostatistics and Medicine, University of California, San Francisco, 550 16th Street, Mission Hall 2nd Floor, San Francisco, CA 94143-0560, USA; [b] Division of General Medicine, Presbyterian Hospital, Columbia University Medical Center, 630 West 168th Street, 9th Floor East, Room 105, New York, NY 10032, USA
* Corresponding author.
E-mail address: mpletcher@epi.ucsf.edu

Med Clin N Am 101 (2017) 673–688
http://dx.doi.org/10.1016/j.mcna.2017.03.002
0025-7125/17/© 2017 Elsevier Inc. All rights reserved.

benefits of the intervention are expected to be large enough to outweigh the cost and risks. In general, persons at very low risk have little to gain from preventive interventions, whereas persons at high risk have much more to gain. As such, cardiovascular risk assessment is critical for effective targeting of CVD prevention interventions to patients most likely to benefit.

Cardiovascular risk assessment has been central to CVD prevention for more than 20 years,[3] and explicitly embedded in guidelines (particularly for cholesterol level–lowering therapy) since the third Adult Treatment Panel (ATP3) guidelines, published in 2001 by the National Cholesterol Education Program.[4] In 2013, the American College of Cardiology (ACC) and American Heart Association (AHA) published guidelines exclusively dedicated to cardiovascular risk assessment methodology.[5] However, cardiovascular risk assessment, remains challenging and controversial. Are clinicians using the right cardiovascular risk factors and the right risk assessment equations and tools? How can clinicians facilitate cardiovascular risk assessment for busy clinical decision makers who are already overwhelmed with information, and help them communicate risk effectively with patients? Can clinicians use genomics, mobile technology, and other biological and technological advancements to improve cardiovascular risk assessment and precise targeting of prevention to high-risk patients who will benefit most? How exactly will cardiovascular risk assessment information be used to guide specific treatment decisions about statins, aspirin, and other preventive interventions?

This article reviews the state of the science of cardiovascular risk assessment with the goal of informing readers about the past, present, and potential future of cardiovascular risk assessment for the purpose of primary prevention of CVD. It covers both practical aspects of risk assessment as well as connections with current thinking on preventive and precision medicine. Although this is not a systematic or comprehensive review of evidence, key references are cited that are either directly useful for clinicians or are illustrative of key concepts, and clinical examples are provided when useful to clarify how the principles of cardiovascular risk assessment may be applied in practice.

THE ROLE OF CARDIOVASCULAR DISEASE RISK ASSESSMENT IN MEDICAL DECISION MAKING
A Brief History of Cardiovascular Risk Assessment

The origins of cardiovascular risk assessment date back to the middle of the twentieth century, when coronary heart disease (CHD) had surged from causing 10% of all deaths in 1900 to about 40% by 1960.[6] As a response to the CHD epidemic, the Framingham Heart Study was organized in 1947 by the US National Heart Institute in the mostly white community of Framingham, Massachusetts, in order to study CVD events in a defined, stable population.[6] In 1960, Framingham investigators introduced the concept of risk factors, observable in the preclinical phase before a first CVD event, that are associated with future cardiovascular risk. Over the next decades, increasing awareness of the risk-multiplying effects (**Fig. 1**) and clustering of multiple risk factors led to development of computational approaches to combining risk factor information about individual patients, and the development of 10-year absolute cardiovascular risk equations designed for routine clinical practice, again pioneered by Framingham investigators and published in 1998.[7] Spurred by the 27th Bethesda Conference,[3] the 2001 National Cholesterol Education Program's ATP3 guideline committee recommended using the Framingham-based 10-year risk equations and an associated Web-based calculator in patients with 2 or more risk factors to decide on thresholds and goals for treatment of low-density lipoprotein (LDL) cholesterol.[4] Although other

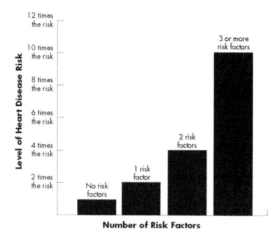

Fig. 1. The multiplier effect of cardiovascular risk factors. Risk for heart disease and other major CVDs increases nonlinearly with increased number of risk factors. Considered here were high blood pressure, high cholesterol level, diabetes, smoking, overweight/obesity, and physical inactivity. (*From* National Heart, Lung, and Blood Institute. Heart disease risk factor "multiplier effect" in midlife women. 2006. Available at: http://www.nhlbi.nih.gov/health/educational/hearttruth/downloads/html/infographic-multiplier/infographic-multiplier.htm. Accessed February 28, 2017; with permission.)

risk assessment tools have been developed subsequently, the Framingham Heart Study established the risk factor concept and the framework for cardiovascular risk assessment for primary prevention, and became the standard against which alternative cardiovascular risk assessment tools are measured.

Traditional Cardiovascular Risk Factors

In the United States and other Western, high-income countries, CHD and other atherosclerotic diseases are the predominant form of CVD. Accordingly, the major traditional risk factors established by the Seven Countries Study,[8] the Framingham Heart Study, and other early cardiovascular epidemiology studies focused on risk factors related to atherosclerosis. This set of major risk factors included age, sex, high total or LDL cholesterol level, low high-density lipoprotein (HDL) cholesterol level, high systolic or diastolic blood pressure, use of antihypertensive medications, diabetes mellitus, tobacco smoking, family history of early CVD, and low socioeconomic status. Of these traditional risk factors, age, sex, blood pressure, lipids, diabetes, and tobacco use are nearly always included in risk assessment algorithms because of their established independent contributions to CVD risk prediction.

Cardiovascular Risk Assessment with Multivariable Risk Equations

The Framingham investigators' approach to combining information from multiple risk factors into an estimate of absolute risk using multivariable risk equations has proved remarkably robust, although it has also been subject to criticism and refinement. One important critique of using Framingham-based equations for cardiovascular risk assessment is the lack of racial–ethnic minority participants in the Framingham cohort. To address this critique, methods for transporting, recalibrating, and validating a cardiovascular risk function (eg, from Framingham) in other

US-based and non–US-based populations have been developed, and these approaches (which generally do not require wholesale refitting of risk equations) have met with some success.[9–11] Several other different risk assessment tools have been developed in other US cohorts that include other racial and ethnic groups, more contemporary data collection, and additional risk factors (**Table 1**). Note that some cardiovascular risk assessment tools require additional testing (eg, C-reactive protein testing for the Reynolds risk functions, coronary artery calcium for the full Multi-Ethnic Study of Atherosclerosis [MESA] risk function), which adds expense and may itself add health risks (eg, radiation from coronary calcium testing). Risk factor and outcome sets vary among these risk functions (see **Table 1**). Cardiovascular risk assessment tools have also been developed for risk assessment in patients in Europe,[12] the United Kingdom,[13] and New Zealand.[14] Despite their differences, the basic approach to risk assessment taken by the Framingham investigators and the core set of risk factors they identified has remained fairly constant.

Of the many multivariable cardiovascular risk assessment tools developed for clinical use, the 2013 ACC/AHA Pooled Cohorts atherosclerotic cardiovascular disease (ASCVD) Risk Equations[5] deserve special mention, because they are currently recommended for use in clinical practice by US national guideline committees[5,15–17]. The Pooled Cohorts ASCVD Risk Equations were derived from a data set of 5 pooled US cardiovascular cohort studies: the ARIC (Atherosclerosis Risk in Communities) Study, the Cardiovascular Health Study, and the CARDIA (Coronary Artery Risk Development in Young Adults) Study, combined with applicable data from the Framingham Original and Offspring Study cohorts, making the estimates statistically robust and allowing derivation of specific equations for African American men, African American women, white men, and white women.[5] Data were insufficient in the Pooled Cohorts data set to support estimates for other race/ethnic groups. Subsequent national guidelines for CVD prevention recommend a central role for cardiovascular risk assessment in guiding interventions, and several now specifically recommend the Pooled Cohorts ASCVD Risk Equations for cardiovascular risk assessment.[15–17]

The Pooled Cohorts Risk Equations have been criticized because many of the data were collected decades ago, and may result in overestimation of risk in contemporary US adults.[18] Risk may be lower in contemporary patients because of lower tobacco smoking intensity compared with past smokers, treatment of increased blood pressure and cholesterol levels earlier in life, and because improved acute treatments (eg, percutaneous coronary intervention) have made acute CVD events less likely to result in severe myocardial infarction or death.[19] Although some validation studies showed reasonable calibration and discrimination of the Pooled Cohorts Risk Equations,[20,21] a recent analyses by Cook and Ridker[22] of the performance of the Pooled Cohorts Risk Equations in 15 external validation cohorts from the United States and Europe suggested that the equations systematically overestimate absolute 10-year cardiovascular risk in many contemporary observational cohorts. Differences between predictions from the Pooled Cohorts Risk Equations and those of other studies may partly be caused by methodological differences between the source studies (eg, method of ascertaining events, see **Table 1**). If the Pooled Cohorts Risk Equations truly overestimate risk, this could lead to substantial overtreatment of low-risk adults. Concern is warranted given the substantial expansion of statin-eligible adults (especially in older adults for whom evidence is sparse) implied by the 2013 cholesterol treatment guidelines.[23]

USING NOVEL RISK FACTORS AND CARDIOVASCULAR DISEASE RISK ASSESSMENT
How Is a Novel Risk Factor Different from a Traditional Risk Factor?

A large body of literature describes novel risk factors or biomarkers for CVD and how they might improve cardiovascular risk assessment and cardiovascular health.[5,24–27] Novel risk factors are distinguished from traditional risk factors by several qualitative differences. Measurements of all traditional risk factors are required for standard cardiovascular risk assessment and are readily available in clinical practice and easy to use without special methods; they can simply be plugged into a standard cardiovascular risk calculator such as the ACC's ASCVD Risk Estimator.[28] In contrast, novel risk factors are not typically ordered, may not be available in all clinical settings, may be more expensive, or may even pose some danger to patients (eg, radiation from measurement of coronary artery calcium level), and are not necessarily easy to incorporate into off-the-shelf risk assessment tools even when the measurement is available. Although special risk calculators[29,30] and other methods[31–34] have been developed to combine information from traditional and novel risk factors, these methods are not widely used or sanctioned by current guidelines. An additional consideration is that many (but not all) traditional risk factors are modifiable causes of disease; in contrast, novel risk factors and biomarkers (as this latter term suggests) are often simply markers of biological processes that predict risk, and are not modifiable treatment targets.

Assessing the Value of a Novel Risk Factor

Given the potential difficulties in obtaining and using novel risk factor measurements, assessing their value to CV risk assessment and CVD prevention is important. Methods for evaluating potential novel risk factors have evolved in recent years. Initial efforts focused on detecting an independent association between the novel risk factor and cardiovascular events after multivariable adjustment for traditional risk factors.[35] Subsequently, focus shifted to use of the C-statistic (ie, area under the receiver-operator characteristic curve) as a metric of improved discrimination between persons who did versus did not go on to develop cardiovascular events.[36] More recently, methods were developed to assess the likelihood of appropriate reclassification across a treatment decision threshold by adding information about the novel risk factor to standard risk assessment using traditional risk factors alone.[37,38] The authors and others have argued that criteria assessing clinical utility of novel risk factors should include metrics of improved health (with or without balancing net effectiveness against costs; ie, cost-effectiveness analysis).[39,40] Note that the value of measuring a novel risk factor is critically dependent on the decision it is meant to influence. For example, the cost-effectiveness of measuring coronary artery calcium level to decide on statin use is much more sensitive to the cost of statins that to the cost of the coronary artery calcium test.[41]

Although methods are still in flux for how to use novel cardiovascular risk factor information, and how to decide which risk factors are worth measuring, the evidence base continues to develop for specific novel cardiovascular risk factors. This evidence has been reviewed recently by a number of guideline committees (**Table 2**), and the US Preventive Services Task Force plans to review this evidence base and update its guideline on risk assessment using nontraditional risk factors in 2018. Evidence specifically supporting the use of markers of subclinical atherosclerosis, serum biomarkers, cumulative exposure measurements, and genetic factors for cardiovascular risk assessment is reviewed here.

Markers of Subclinical Atherosclerosis

The strongest novel predictors of atherosclerotic CVD events are indicators of the presence and extent of subclinical atherosclerosis. Atherosclerosis can be

Table 1
Ten-year cardiovascular disease risk functions generated from United States cohort studies

10-y Risk Prediction Function	FRS-CHD	ATPIII-FRS-CHD	Reynolds Risk Score for Women	Reynolds Risk Score for Men	FRS-CVD	AHA-ACC-ASCVD	MESA Risk Function	JHS (Model 1)
Year/Reference	1998[7]	2002[7,79]	2007[80]	2008[81]	2008[82]	2014[5,83]	2015[84]	2016[85]
Cohort at Baseline (N)	5345	5345	24,558 (Women's Health Study)	10,724 (Physicians Health Study II)	8491	24,626	6814	3689
Race/Ethnic Makeup at Baseline	Predominantly white	Predominantly white	Included white, black, Hispanic, Asian, other, but not used in calibration	—	Predominantly white	White, black	White, black, Hispanic, Asian	Black
Baseline Year	1971–1974	1971–1974	1992	1995	1968–1971 1971–1975 1984–1987	—	2000–2002	2000–2004
CVD Outcomes	• CHD death • Nonfatal MI • Unstable angina • Stable angina	• CHD death • Nonfatal MI	• Cardiovascular death • Nonfatal MI • Nonfatal stroke • Coronary revascularization	• Cardiovascular death • Nonfatal MI • Nonfatal stroke • Coronary revascularization	• CHD death • Nonfatal MI • Coronary insufficiency or angina • Fatal or nonfatal ischemic or hemorrhagic stroke • Transient ischemic attack • Intermittent claudication • Heart failure	• CHD death • Nonfatal MI • Fatal stroke • Nonfatal stroke	• CHD death • Nonfatal MI • Resuscitated cardiac arrest • Coronary revascularization in patient with angina	• MI • Fatal CHD • Heart failure • Stroke • Angina • Claudication

Risk Factors in Risk Function							
• Age • Gender • Total C or LDL-C (mg/dL) • HDL-C (mg/dL) • SBP (mm Hg) • Diabetes mellitus (yes or no) • Current smoking (yes or no)	• Age • Gender • Total C (mg/dL) • HDL-C (mg/dL) • SBP (mm Hg) • BP treatment (yes or no) • Current smoking (yes or no)	• Age • Total C (mg/dL) • HDL-C (mg/dL) • SBP (mm Hg) • Diabetes mellitus assessed by hemoglobin A1c (%) • Current smoking (yes or no) • Parental history of MI before age 60 y (yes or no) • Serum hs-CRP (mg/L)	• Age • Total C (mg/dL) • HDL-C (mg/dL) • SBP (mm Hg) • Current smoking (yes or no) • Parental history of MI before age 60 y (yes or no) • Serum hs-CRP (mg/L)	• Age • Gender • Total C (mg/dL) • HDL-C (mg/dL) • SBP (mm Hg) • BP treatment (yes or no) • Diabetes mellitus (yes or no) • Current smoking (yes or no)	• Age • Gender • Total C (mg/dL) • HDL-C (mg/dL) • SBP (mm Hg) • BP treatment (yes or no) • Diabetes mellitus (yes or no) • Current smoking (yes or no)	• Age • Gender • Ethnicity (non-Hispanic white, Chinese American, African American, Hispanic) • Total C (mg/dL) • HDL-C (mg/dL) • Lipid level–lowering treatment (yes or no) • SBP (mm Hg) • BP treatment (yes or no) • Diabetes mellitus (yes or no) • Current smoking (yes or no) • Family history of MI at any age (yes or no) • Coronary artery calcium score	• Age • Gender • BMI • SBP • BP Treatment • Diabetes mellitus (yes or no) • Ratio of total C to HDL-C (mg/dL) • Current smoking (yes or no) • eGFR (CKD-EPI equation)

Abbreviations: ASCVD, atherosclerotic cardiovascular disease; BMI, body mass index; BP, blood pressure; C, cholesterol; CKD-EPI, Chronic Kidney Disease Epidemiology Collaboration; eGFR, estimated glomerular filtration rate; FRS, Framingham Risk Score; HDL-C, high-density lipoprotein cholesterol; hs-CRP, high-sensitivity C-reactive protein; JHS, Jackson Heart Study; LDL-C, low-density lipoprotein cholesterol; MESA, Multi-Ethnic Study of Atherosclerosis; MI, myocardial infarction; SBP, systolic blood pressure.

Table 2
Novel cardiovascular risk factors reviewed and recommended (X) or Not (−) by different guideline committees

Novel Risk Factor	2009 and 2013 US Preventive Services Task Force[24,86]	2013 ACC/AHA Guidelines[5,16]	2016 European Guidelines on CVD Prevention[27]
Coronary artery calcium	−	X	X
Carotid intima media thickness	−	−	−
Carotid plaque detection	NR	NR	X
Ankle-brachial index	−	X	X
C-reactive protein	−	X	−
Lipoprotein (a)	−	NR	NR
Homocysteine	−	NR	−
Leukocyte count	−	NR	NR
Fasting blood glucose	−	NR	−
Apolipoprotein B	NR	−	NR
Lipoprotein-associated phospholipase A2	NR	NR	−
Genetic factors	NR	NR	−
Family history	NR	X	X
Social factors	NR	NR	X
Obesity	NR	NR	X
Cardiovascular fitness	NR	−	NR
Periodontal disease	−	NR	−
Chronic kidney disease, low glomerular filtration rate, or microalbuminuria	NR	−	−
Rheumatoid arthritis or other autoimmune disease	NR	NR	X

The symbol "X" indicates a novel risk factor recommended for use in the specified guideline. "−" indicates a novel risk factor specifically reviewed and not recommended for use in the specified guideline.
Abbreviation: NR, not specifically reviewed.

detected, for example, in the descending aorta/periphery by measurement of the ankle-brachial index, in carotid arteries by ultrasonography-based assessment of carotid artery intima media thickness, or in the coronary arteries by computed tomography–based detection and quantification of coronary artery calcium (CAC). Of these, the most established and strongest predictor is CAC. A standard protocol is available for measuring the CAC score,[42] which is independently associated with major coronary events (relative risks of 3–7 comparing moderate/high levels with zero),[43] measurably improves discrimination (C-statistic, 0.79 improved to 0.83; $P = .006$),[43] leads to substantial net reclassification improvement,[44] can be integrated with traditional risk factors using published methods to obtain an updated risk estimate,[32] is cost-effective to measure in limited circumstances,[41] and is recommended as a secondary risk assessment factor that can be used to inform treatment decision making,[5] in particular regarding cholesterol treatment decisions.[16] The ankle-brachial index is a weaker predictor, but because of its ease of measurement, it is also recognized as a reasonable secondary risk assessment factor[5]; other subclinical measures, including the carotid intima media thickness, are not recommended for routine measurement.[5]

Serum Biomarkers

Blood testing, which is required for measurement of total, LDL, and HDL cholesterol, already plays an important role in cardiovascular risk assessment. It may therefore be efficient to perform additional tests if those tests provide information useful for risk stratification. The best established novel risk factor measurable through blood testing is high-sensitivity C-reactive protein, which is independently associated with CVD events,[45] leads to significant reclassification improvement,[38,46] and is recommended as a secondary risk assessment factor that can inform treatment decision making,[5] in particular with regard to treatment of blood cholesterol.[16] However, the C-reactive protein assay is expensive, and there is some doubt that C-reactive protein testing is a cost-effective means of guiding preventive therapy.[47] Many other serum biomarkers have been found to be independently associated with CVD events, including other markers of inflammation (interleukin-6, Lipoprotein-associated phospholipase A2 [lpPLA2]), oxidative stress (oxidized LDL, nitrotyrosine), lipid metabolism [lipoprotein (a)], thrombosis (plasminogen activator inhibitor-1, D-dimer), endothelial dysfunction (homocysteine, urinary microalbuminuria), hemodynamic stress (natriuretic peptides), cardiomyocyte injury (cardiac troponins),[48] and hyperglycemia (hemoglobin A1c or fasting blood sugar),[49] but evidence that these biomarkers improve reclassification or otherwise improve decision making or outcomes is limited,[34,48,49] and no serum biomarkers other than C-reactive protein were recommended for preventive treatment decision making in recent reviews.[5,16,24]

Genetic Risk Factors

Large-scale genome-wide association studies have identified many single-nucleotide polymorphisms (SNPs) and multi-SNP genetic risk scores that are independently associated with CVD events.[50–53] Genetic risk factors are not strong predictors of events (relative risks, <2), but have recently been shown to improve discrimination and reclassification to some degree.[53] Recent guidelines and reviews do not address genetic risk factors,[5,24] and few cost-effectiveness or decision analyses have been performed to quantify the potential benefits in terms of clinical outcomes that might result from use of genetic information for cardiovascular risk assessment.[53–55] An exception may be genetic testing for familial hypercholesterolemia, which can help identify individuals (and their family members) at high cardiovascular risk who could potentially benefit from cholesterol level–lowering therapy[56]; but no direct evidence yet supports a health benefit from screening.[57]

FUTURE OF CARDIOVASCULAR DISEASE RISK ASSESSMENT
Decision Support for Cardiovascular Disease Risk Assessment

Busy clinicians need ways to expedite the calculations and shared decision making they must accomplish, usually during clinic visits, to incorporate cardiovascular risk assessment into their patient care routines. User-friendly tools exist to facilitate calculation of cardiovascular risk (eg, the ACC ASCVD Risk Estimator[28]) and help patients understand the potential benefits of statin therapy.[58] Risk estimation tools are now being built into electronic health record systems that will automatically extract the required clinical measurements and estimate risk.[59,60] The nature of clinical measurements such as blood pressure (repeated, noisy and error-prone, often missing and asynchronous with other risk factor measurements) poses challenges to these methods, but surfacing and addressing these issues directly and scientifically will facilitate implementation of risk prediction into clinical practice so that scientific advancements in cardiovascular risk assessment can effectively translate into improved decision making for providers and improved health for patients.

Lifetime Risk Versus 10-year Risk

Most risk equations estimate 10-year risk, which is an intuitive time frame that resonates with patients and clinicians who use risk estimates for practical decision making. However, this time frame may be too short to capture long-term effects of risk factors and preventive interventions, and it strongly emphasizes the impact of increasing age on cardiovascular risk, which is nonmodifiable. For example, young adulthood may be a critical time to focus on risk factor control, because keeping risk factors in an ideal range through young adulthood is independently associated with lower event rates later in life[61,62]; however, a focus on 10-year risk never emphasizes risk factor control in young adults, because 10-year risk is universally low during this time. Methods for estimating lifetime cardiovascular risk have been developed,[63] may help inform patient-clinician communications,[64] and could theoretically lead to different decision making about use of preventive medications early in life.[65,66] A randomized trial testing the effectiveness of statin therapy for young adults (men 35–50 years of age, and women 45–59 years of age) with low short-term risk but high lifetime risk is currently underway.[67]

Absolute Risk Reduction Versus Baseline Risk

The premise of cardiovascular risk assessment is that baseline cardiovascular risk is the key to efficient and effective targeting of preventive treatments like statins, because baseline cardiovascular risk is a good surrogate measure for the potential benefit that individuals might obtain from a preventive treatment. Implicit in this strategy is that all individuals for whom the preventive treatment is being considered obtain the same relative risk reduction from that treatment. However, there is evidence that statin efficacy (in terms of relative risk reduction) may be higher in individuals with higher baseline LDL levels and younger age,[68,69] higher C-reactive protein levels,[70] or with higher genetic risk scores[52] (although recent evidence does not necessarily support this heterogeneity[71]). If these characteristics modify the effectiveness of statins, then clinicians should directly estimate expected absolute risk reduction from statin therapy, accounting for these individual characteristics, before a prescription is written (eg, benefit-targeted prevention, rather than risk-targeted prevention[69,72]). This precision medicine approach to targeting preventive therapy could provide substantial benefits for individuals who, for example, can avoid a lifetime of statin use if it is known that it will provide negligible benefit.[69,72] However, translating this approach into clinical practice requires the production of reproducible quantitative methods for estimating expected individual-level absolute risk reduction with treatment,[69] as well as absolute risk reduction calculators and decision support tools that can be used at the point of care.

Using Cardiovascular Disease Risk Assessment for Guiding Hypertension Treatment

Cardiovascular risk assessment has been recommended for guiding cholesterol level–lowering treatment since 2001,[4] and for aspirin since 2002.[73] Cardiovascular risk assessment could also guide hypertension treatment, as has recently been argued[74] (the same basic rationale holds), and modeling efforts suggest that risk-based treatment would be more efficient.[75] The Systolic Blood Pressure Treatment Trial (SPRINT) found that intensive systolic blood pressure treatment reduced cardiovascular risk and all-cause mortality in patients with high cardiovascular risk,[76] but it remains less clear that intensive treatment benefits extend to patients with intermediate cardiovascular risk.[77] In any case, guidelines to date have recommended treatment of hypertension with medications based on blood pressure levels rather than on cardiovascular risk.[78] A counter-rationale in favor of blood pressure level–based prescribing not currently accounted for in modeling studies is that cumulative irreversible damage from high blood pressure levels early in life could occur if clinicians wait to prescribe hypertensive medications until cardiovascular risk increases above some threshold. New evidence supports this counter-rationale,[61] but the issue is far from settled. New US hypertension guidelines due out in the next year or so will be the first to account for results from SPRINT, and will likely address the question of cardiovascular risk–based hypertension treatment.

SUMMARY AND FUTURE CONSIDERATIONS

Cardiovascular risk assessment has been a mainstay of cardiovascular risk prevention efforts since the mid–twentieth century, and remains an active area of research. Recent efforts are designed to improve risk prediction by pooling data from multiple cohorts, considering the addition of novel risk factors like C-reactive protein and CAC, and advancing methods for estimating the value of measuring novel risk factors. However, the basic rubric persists: assess cardiovascular risk, and target preventive therapy preferentially to persons at higher risk because they have more to gain from that therapy. The authors believe that the future will bring incremental improvements in risk prediction through genetics, data mining, use of the predicted absolute risk reduction instead of the predictive baseline risk for guiding preventive therapy, and better incorporation of automated risk calculators and decision aids into electronic health record platforms for ease of use by clinicians at the point of care. Although debate and controversy about how to approach cardiovascular risk assessment are not over, it is worth celebrating advances in cardiovascular risk assessment science, the key role risk assessment now plays in CVD prevention guidelines, the broad clinical adoption of cardiovascular risk assessment tools for medical decision making, and the likely role that cardiovascular risk assessment has played in the decades-long declines seen in CVD mortality achieved in the US population.[1]

REFERENCES

1. Mozaffarian D, Benjamin EJ, Go AS, et al. Heart disease and stroke statistics-2016 update: a report from the American Heart Association. Circulation 2016; 133(4):e38–360.
2. Mozaffarian D, Wilson PW, Kannel WB. Beyond established and novel risk factors: lifestyle risk factors for cardiovascular disease. Circulation 2008;117(23): 3031–8.
3. 27th Bethesda Conference. Matching the intensity of risk factor management with the hazard for coronary disease events. September 14-15, 1995. J Am Coll Cardiol 1996;27(5):957–1047.
4. Expert Panel on Detection, Evaluation, and Treatment of High Blood Cholesterol in Adults. Executive summary of the third report of the National Cholesterol Education Program (NCEP) Expert Panel on Detection, Evaluation, and Treatment of High Blood Cholesterol in Adults (Adult Treatment Panel III). JAMA 2001;285(19): 2486–97.
5. Goff DC Jr, Lloyd-Jones DM, Bennett G, et al. 2013 ACC/AHA guideline on the assessment of cardiovascular risk: a report of the American College of

Cardiology/American Heart Association Task Force on Practice Guidelines. Circulation 2014;129(25 Suppl 2):S49–73.

6. Wong ND, Levy D. Legacy of the Framingham Heart Study: rationale, design, initial findings, and implications. Glob Heart 2013;8(1):3–9.

7. Wilson PW, D'Agostino RB, Levy D, et al. Prediction of coronary heart disease using risk factor categories. Circulation 1998;97(18):1837–47.

8. Menotti A, Keys A, Blackburn H, et al. Comparison of multivariate predictive power of major risk factors for coronary heart diseases in different countries: results from eight nations of the Seven Countries Study, 25-year follow-up. J Cardiovasc Risk 1996;3(1):69–75.

9. D'Agostino RB, Grundy S, Sullivan LM, et al. Validation of the Framingham coronary heart disease prediction scores. JAMA 2001;286:180–7.

10. Liu J, Hong Y, D'Agostino RB, et al. Predictive value for the Chinese population of the Framingham CHD risk assessment tool compared with the Chinese Multi-Provincial Cohort Study. JAMA 2004;291(21):2591–9.

11. Wu Y, Liu X, Li X, et al. Estimation of 10-year risk of fatal and nonfatal ischemic cardiovascular diseases in Chinese adults. Circulation 2006;114(21):2217–25.

12. Conroy RM, Pyorala K, Fitzgerald AP, et al. Estimation of ten-year risk of fatal cardiovascular disease in Europe: the SCORE project. Eur Heart J 2003;24(11): 987–1003.

13. Hippisley-Cox J, Coupland C, Vinogradova Y, et al. Predicting cardiovascular risk in England and Wales: prospective derivation and validation of QRISK2. BMJ 2008;336(7659):1475–82.

14. Bannink L, Wells S, Broad J, et al. Web-based assessment of cardiovascular disease risk in routine primary care practice in New Zealand: the first 18,000 patients (PREDICT CVD-1). N Z Med J 2006;119(1245):U2313.

15. US Preventive Services Task Force, Bibbins-Domingo K, Grossman DC, Curry SJ, et al. Statin use for the primary prevention of cardiovascular disease in adults: US Preventive Services Task Force recommendation statement. JAMA 2016;316(19): 1997–2007.

16. Stone NJ, Robinson J, Lichtenstein AH, et al. 2013 ACC/AHA guideline on the treatment of blood cholesterol to reduce atherosclerotic cardiovascular risk in adults: a report of the American College of Cardiology/American Heart Association Task Force on Practice Guidelines. Circulation 2014;129(25 Suppl 2):S1–45.

17. Bibbins-Domingo K, U.S. Preventive Services Task Force. Aspirin use for the primary prevention of cardiovascular disease and colorectal cancer: U.S. Preventive Services Task Force recommendation statement. Ann Intern Med 2016; 164(12):836–45.

18. Ridker PM, Cook NR. Statins: new American guidelines for prevention of cardiovascular disease. Lancet 2013;382(9907):1762–5.

19. Muntner P, Safford MM, Cushman M, et al. Comment on the reports of overestimation of ASCVD risk using the 2013 AHA/ACC risk equation. Circulation 2014;129(2):266–7.

20. Muntner P, Colantonio LD, Cushman M, et al. Validation of the atherosclerotic cardiovascular disease pooled cohort risk equations. JAMA 2014;311(14):1406–15.

21. Mortensen MB, Afzal S, Nordestgaard BG, et al. Primary prevention with statins: ACC/AHA risk-based approach versus trial-based approaches to guide statin therapy. J Am Coll Cardiol 2015;66(24):2699–709.

22. Cook NR, Ridker PM. Calibration of the pooled cohort equations for atherosclerotic cardiovascular disease: an update. Ann Intern Med 2016;165(11):786–94.

23. Pencina MJ, Navar-Boggan AM, D'Agostino RB Sr, et al. Application of new cholesterol guidelines to a population-based sample. N Engl J Med 2014; 370(15):1422–31.
24. Helfand M, Buckley DI, Freeman M, et al. Emerging risk factors for coronary heart disease: a summary of systematic reviews conducted for the U.S. Preventive Services Task Force. Ann Intern Med 2009;151(7):496–507.
25. Wang TJ, Gona P, Larson MG, et al. Multiple biomarkers for the prediction of first major cardiovascular events and death. N Engl J Med 2006;355(25):2631–9.
26. Yeboah J, McClelland RL, Polonsky TS, et al. Comparison of novel risk markers for improvement in cardiovascular risk assessment in intermediate-risk individuals. JAMA 2012;308(8):788–95.
27. Piepoli MF, Hoes AW, Agewall S, et al. 2016 European guidelines on cardiovascular disease prevention in clinical practice: The Sixth Joint Task Force of the European Society of Cardiology and Other Societies on Cardiovascular Disease Prevention in Clinical Practice (constituted by representatives of 10 societies and by invited experts). Developed with the special contribution of the European Association for Cardiovascular Prevention & Rehabilitation (EACPR). Eur Heart J 2016;37(29):2315–81.
28. American College of Cardiology. ASCVD risk estimator. Available at: http://tools. acc.org/ASCVD-Risk-Estimator/. Accessed April 2, 2017.
29. Reynolds Risk Score. Available at: http://www.reynoldsriskscore.org/. Accessed April 2, 2017.
30. MESA. MESA 10-year CHD risk with coronary artery calcification. Available at: https://www.mesa-nhlbi.org/MESACHDRisk/MesaRiskScore/RiskScore.aspx. Accessed April 2, 2017.
31. Kooter AJ, Kostense PJ, Groenewold J, et al. Integrating information from novel risk factors with calculated risks: the critical impact of risk factor prevalence. Circulation 2011;124(6):741–5.
32. Pletcher MJ, Sibley C, Pignone M, et al. Interpretation of the coronary artery calcium score in combination with conventional cardiovascular risk factors: the Multi-ethnic Study of Atherosclerosis (MESA). Circulation 2013;128(10):1076–84.
33. Pletcher MJ, Tice JA, Pignone M, et al. What does my patient's coronary artery calcium score mean? Combining information from the coronary artery calcium score with information from conventional risk factors to estimate coronary heart disease risk. BMC Med 2004;2(1):31.
34. Jarmul JA, Pignone M, Pletcher MJ. Interpreting hemoglobin A1C in combination with conventional risk factors for prediction of cardiovascular risk. Circ Cardiovasc Qual Outcomes 2015;8(5):501–7.
35. Ridker PM, Hennekens CH, Buring JE, et al. C-reactive protein and other markers of inflammation in the prediction of cardiovascular disease in women. N Engl J Med 2000;342(12):836–43.
36. Zou KH, O'Malley AJ, Mauri L. Receiver-operating characteristic analysis for evaluating diagnostic tests and predictive models. Circulation 2007;115(5):654–7.
37. Pencina MJ, D'Agostino RB Sr, D'Agostino RB Jr, et al. Evaluating the added predictive ability of a new marker: from area under the ROC curve to reclassification and beyond. Stat Med 2008;27(2):157–72 [discussion: 207–12].
38. Cook NR, Buring JE, Ridker PM. The effect of including C-reactive protein in cardiovascular risk prediction models for women. Ann Intern Med 2006;145(1):21–9.
39. Pletcher MJ, Pignone M. Evaluating the clinical utility of a biomarker: a review of methods for estimating health impact. Circulation 2011;123(10):1116–24.

40. Hlatky MA, Greenland P, Arnett DK, et al. Criteria for evaluation of novel markers of cardiovascular risk: a scientific statement from the American Heart Association. Circulation 2009;119(17):2408–16.

41. Pletcher MJ, Pignone M, Earnshaw S, et al. Using the coronary artery calcium score to guide statin therapy: a cost-effectiveness analysis. Circ Cardiovasc Qual Outcomes 2014;7(2):276–84.

42. Agatston AS, Janowitz WR, Hildner FJ, et al. Quantification of coronary artery calcium using ultrafast computed tomography. J Am Coll Cardiol 1990;15(4): 827–32.

43. Detrano R, Guerci AD, Carr JJ, et al. Coronary calcium as a predictor of coronary events in four racial or ethnic groups. N Engl J Med 2008;358(13):1336–45.

44. Polonsky TS, McClellan RL, Jorgensen NW, et al. Coronary artery calcium score and risk classification for coronary heart disease prediction. JAMA 2010;303(16): 1610–6.

45. Buckley DI, Fu R, Freeman M, et al. C-reactive protein as a risk factor for coronary heart disease: a systematic review and meta-analyses for the U.S. Preventive Services Task Force. Ann Intern Med 2009;151(7):483–95.

46. Wilson PW, Pencina M, Jacques P, et al. C-reactive protein and reclassification of cardiovascular risk in the Framingham Heart Study. Circ Cardiovasc Qual Outcomes 2008;1(2):92–7.

47. Lee KK, Cipriano LE, Owens DK, et al. Cost-effectiveness of using high-sensitivity C-reactive protein to identify intermediate- and low-cardiovascular-risk individuals for statin therapy. Circulation 2010;122(15):1478–87.

48. Wang TJ. Assessing the role of circulating, genetic, and imaging biomarkers in cardiovascular risk prediction. Circulation 2011;123(5):551–65.

49. Selvin E, Steffes MW, Zhu H, et al. Glycated hemoglobin, diabetes, and cardiovascular risk in nondiabetic adults. N Engl J Med 2010;362(9):800–11.

50. Roberts R, Stewart AF. Genes and coronary artery disease: where are we? J Am Coll Cardiol 2012;60(18):1715–21.

51. Deloukas P, Kanoni S, Willenborg C, et al. Large-scale association analysis identifies new risk loci for coronary artery disease. Nat Genet 2013;45(1):25–33.

52. Mega JL, Stitziel NO, Smith JG, et al. Genetic risk, coronary heart disease events, and the clinical benefit of statin therapy: an analysis of primary and secondary prevention trials. Lancet 2015;385(9984):2264–71.

53. Iribarren C, Lu M, Jorgenson E, et al. Clinical utility of multi-marker genetic risk scores for prediction of incident coronary heart disease: a cohort study among over 51 thousand individuals of European ancestry. Circ Cardiovasc Genet 2016;9(6):531–40.

54. Ademi Z, Watts GF, Pang J, et al. Cascade screening based on genetic testing is cost-effective: evidence for the implementation of models of care for familial hypercholesterolemia. J Clin Lipidol 2014;8(4):390–400.

55. Ramirez de Arellano A, Coca A, de la Figuera M, et al. Economic evaluation of Cardio inCode®, a clinical-genetic function for coronary heart disease risk assessment. Appl Health Econ Health Policy 2013;11(5):531–42.

56. Wald DS, Bestwick JP, Morris JK, et al. Child-parent familial hypercholesterolemia screening in primary care. N Engl J Med 2016;375(17):1628–37.

57. Lozano P, Henrikson NB, Morrison CC, et al. Lipid screening in childhood and adolescence for detection of multifactorial dyslipidemia: evidence report and systematic review for the US preventive services task force. JAMA 2016;316(6): 634–44.

58. Statin Choice: Decision Aid. Available at: https://statindecisionaid.mayoclinic.org/. Accessed April 2, 2017.

59. Gluckman TJ. The ACC/AHA ASCVD risk estimator app and the EHR FHIR integration project. Available at: https://www.himssconference.org/sites/himssconference/files/pdf/IS22.pdf. Accessed April 2, 2017.

60. Pike MM, Decker PA, Larson NB, et al. Improvement in cardiovascular risk prediction with electronic health records. J Cardiovasc Transl Res 2016;9(3):214–22.

61. Pletcher MJ, Vittinghoff E, Thanataveerat A, et al. Young adult exposure to cardiovascular risk factors and risk of events later in life: the Framingham Offspring Study. PLoS One 2016;11(5):e0154288.

62. Stamler J, Stamler R, Neaton JD, et al. Low risk-factor profile and long-term cardiovascular and noncardiovascular mortality and life expectancy: findings for 5 large cohorts of young adult and middle-aged men and women. JAMA 1999; 282(21):2012–8.

63. Berry JD, Dyer A, Cai X, et al. Lifetime risks of cardiovascular disease. N Engl J Med 2012;366(4):321–9.

64. Karmali KN, Lloyd-Jones DM. Adding a life-course perspective to cardiovascular-risk communication. Nat Rev Cardiol 2013;10(2):111–5.

65. Pletcher MJ, Hulley SB. Statin prescribing in young adults: ready for prime time? J Am Coll Cardiol 2010;56(8):637–40.

66. Steinberg D. Earlier intervention in the management of hypercholesterolemia: what are we waiting for? J Am Coll Cardiol 2010;56(8):627–9.

67. Domanski MJ, Fuster V, Diaz-Mitoma F, et al. Next steps in primary prevention of coronary heart disease: rationale for and design of the ECAD trial. J Am Coll Cardiol 2015;66(16):1828–36.

68. Mihaylova B, Emberson J, Blackwell L, et al. The effects of lowering LDL cholesterol with statin therapy in people at low risk of vascular disease: meta-analysis of individual data from 27 randomised trials. Lancet 2012;380(9841):581–90.

69. Thanassoulis G, Williams K, Kimler Altobelli K, et al. Individualized statin benefit for determining statin eligibility in the primary prevention of cardiovascular disease. Circulation 2016;133(16):1574–81.

70. Ridker PM, Rifai N, Clearfield M, et al. Measurement of C-reactive protein for the targeting of statin therapy in the primary prevention of acute coronary events. N Engl J Med 2001;344(26):1959–65.

71. Yusuf S, Bosch J, Dagenais G, et al. Cholesterol lowering in intermediate-risk persons without cardiovascular disease. N Engl J Med 2016;374(21):2021–31.

72. Pletcher MJ, Pignone M, Jarmul JA, et al. Population impact and efficiency of benefit-targeted vs. risk-targeted statin prescribing for primary prevention of cardiovascular disease. J Am Heart Assoc 2017;6(2):2.

73. U.S. Preventive Services Task Force. Aspirin for the primary prevention of cardiovascular events: recommendation and rationale. Ann Intern Med 2002;136(2): 157–60.

74. Navar AM, Pencina MJ, Peterson ED. Assessing cardiovascular risk to guide hypertension diagnosis and treatment. JAMA Cardiol 2016;1(8):864–71.

75. Sussman J, Vijan S, Hayward R. Using benefit-based tailored treatment to improve the use of antihypertensive medications. Circulation 2013;128(21): 2309–17.

76. Group SR, Wright JT Jr, Williamson JD, et al. A randomized trial of intensive versus standard blood-pressure control. N Engl J Med 2015;373(22):2103–16.

77. Lonn EM, Bosch J, Lopez-Jaramillo P, et al. Blood-pressure lowering in intermediate-risk persons without cardiovascular disease. N Engl J Med 2016; 374(21):2009–20.

78. Go AS, Bauman MA, Coleman King SM, et al. An effective approach to high blood pressure control: a science advisory from the American Heart Association, the American College of Cardiology, and the Centers for Disease Control and Prevention. Hypertension 2014;63(4):878–85.

79. National Cholesterol Education Program (NCEP) Expert Panel on Detection, Evaluation, and Treatment of High Blood Cholesterol in Adults (Adult Treatment Panel III). Third report of the National Cholesterol Education Program (NCEP) Expert Panel on Detection, Evaluation, and Treatment of High Blood Cholesterol in Adults (Adult Treatment Panel III) final report. Circulation 2002;106(25):3143–421.

80. Ridker PM, Buring JE, Rifai N, et al. Development and validation of improved algorithms for the assessment of global cardiovascular risk in women: the Reynolds Risk Score. JAMA 2007;297(6):611–9.

81. Ridker PM, Paynter NP, Rifai N, et al. C-reactive protein and parental history improve global cardiovascular risk prediction: the Reynolds Risk Score for men. Circulation 2008;118(22):2243–51, 4p following 51.

82. D'Agostino RB Sr, Vasan RS, Pencina MJ, et al. General cardiovascular risk profile for use in primary care: the Framingham Heart Study. Circulation 2008;117(6): 743–53.

83. Karmali KN, Goff DC Jr, Ning H, et al. A systematic examination of the 2013 ACC/AHA pooled cohort risk assessment tool for atherosclerotic cardiovascular disease. J Am Coll Cardiol 2014;64(10):959–68.

84. McClelland RL, Jorgensen NW, Budoff M, et al. 10-year coronary heart disease risk prediction using coronary artery calcium and traditional risk factors: derivation in the MESA (Multi-ethnic Study of Atherosclerosis) with validation in the HNR (Heinz Nixdorf Recall) study and the DHS (Dallas Heart Study). J Am Coll Cardiol 2015;66(15):1643–53.

85. Fox ER, Samdarshi TE, Musani SK, et al. Development and validation of risk prediction models for cardiovascular events in black adults: the Jackson Heart Study cohort. JAMA Cardiol 2016;1(1):15–25.

86. Moyer VA, US Preventive Services Task Force. Screening for peripheral artery disease and cardiovascular disease risk assessment with the ankle-brachial index in adults: U.S. Preventive Services Task Force recommendation statement. Ann Intern Med 2013;159(5):342–8.

Statins for Primary Prevention of Cardiovascular Disease

Review of Evidence and Recommendations for Clinical Practice

Dhruv S. Kazi, MD, MSc, MS[a,b,c,d,e], Joanne M. Penko, MS, MPH[c,f],
Kirsten Bibbins-Domingo, PhD, MD, MAS[a,b,c,f,*]

KEYWORDS

- Cholesterol • Statin • 10-year risk • Cardiovascular disease • Lipids
- Statin intolerance

KEY POINTS

- Large clinical trials have shown statin therapy to be effective and safe for primary prevention of atherosclerotic cardiovascular disease (CVD) for adults age 40 to 75 years.
- Online 10-year CVD risk calculators can help define eligibility for statin therapy.
- Statin treatment for primary prevention in adults older than 75 years remains uncertain due to sparse research evidence.
- Despite high-quality evidence of effectiveness, safety, and cost-effectiveness, statins are underutilized for primary prevention.
- Decisions around initiation of statin therapy with individual patients should include discussions of benefits and risks of treatment, lifestyle changes, and plans for monitoring for side effects.

Disclosure Statement: The authors have no disclosures to report.
[a] Department of Medicine, University of California San Francisco, 505 Parnassus Avenue, San Francisco, CA 94122, USA; [b] Department of Epidemiology, University of California San Francisco, 550 16th Street, San Francisco, CA 94158, USA; [c] UCSF Center for Vulnerable Populations, 2789 25th Street, Suite 350, San Francisco, CA 94110, USA; [d] UCSF Center for Healthcare Value, 3333 California Street, Suite 265, San Francisco, CA 94118, USA; [e] Division of Cardiology, Zuckerberg San Francisco General Hospital, 1001 Potrero Avenue, San Francisco, CA 94110, USA; [f] Division of General Internal Medicine, Zuckerberg San Francisco General Hospital, UCSF Box 1364, San Francisco, CA 94143-1364, USA
* Corresponding author. UCSF Box 1364, San Francisco, CA 94143-1364.
E-mail address: kirsten.bibbins-domingo@ucsf.edu

Med Clin N Am 101 (2017) 689–699
http://dx.doi.org/10.1016/j.mcna.2017.03.001
0025-7125/17/© 2017 Elsevier Inc. All rights reserved.

medical.theclinics.com

INTRODUCTION

Cardiovascular disease (CVD) remains a leading cause of morbidity and mortality in the United States despite steady improvements over the past several decades.[1] High serum cholesterol, specifically low-density lipoprotein cholesterol (LDL-C), is associated with an increased risk of atherosclerotic CVD. LDL-C reduction with statin therapy has been a cornerstone of CVD prevention since the introduction of statin medications in the late 1980s.[1] Statins are a class of lipid-lowering agents that inhibit the enzyme 3-hydroxy-3-methyl-glutaryl coenzyme A reductase, which catalyzes a rate-limiting step in cholesterol production. Treatment with statins leads to reduced serum levels of total cholesterol, LDL-C, and triglycerides.[2] Seven statin drugs are currently available in the United States and are categorized according to the degree of effect on LDL-C levels: (1) low-intensity statins lower LDL-C by less than 30%; (2) moderate-intensity statins lower LDL-C by 30% to 50%; and (3) high-intensity statins lower LDL-C by 50% or more.

The purpose of this review is both to present the current state of research on statin use in adults for primary prevention of incident atherosclerotic CVD and to provide practical advice for prescribing statins among patients without preexisting atherosclerotic CVD in general medicine practice. In particular, the article focuses on recent reviews of evidence and guidelines from the American College of Cardiology/American Heart Association (ACC/AHA) and the US Preventive Services Task Force (USPSTF).[2,3] Although differing in many specifics, both define the primary prevention target population and statin dosing based on calculations of patients' 10-year risk of having an atherosclerotic CVD event, departing from prior approaches that recommended use of statins to treat populations above certain threshold LDL-C levels. The authors highlight the rationale for this approach as well as address several areas of uncertainty.

EVIDENCE OF EFFICACY, SAFETY, AND COST-EFFECTIVENESS
Statins Are Effective for Primary Prevention of Atherosclerotic Cardiovascular Disease

A large body of evidence from high-quality randomized clinical trials indicates that statins are effective at reducing levels of serum LDL-C and total cholesterol as well as the risk of vascular events and deaths.[4–6] A recent systematic review, commissioned by the USPSTF to inform their guidelines, evaluated evidence from randomized trials comparing statins to placebo in adults older than 40 years of age without a history of atherosclerotic CVD.[4] The review included 19 randomized clinical trials that followed patients for coronary heart disease, stroke, and/or all-cause mortality for up to 6 years. All trials enrolled patients with one or more risk factors for atherosclerotic CVD: one-third used dyslipidemia as the main eligibility criterion; others selected patients based on other atherosclerotic CVD risk factors such as diabetes, hypertension, or early cerebrovascular disease.

In these studies, patients randomized to receiving statins compared with placebo had a 30% decreased risk of adverse cardiovascular outcomes (relative risk [RR] = 0.70, 95% confidence interval [CI]: 0.63–0.78) and a 14% decreased risk of all-cause mortality (RR = 0.86, 95% CI: 0.80–0.93).[4] Patients randomized to statins experienced fewer myocardial infarctions (RR = 0.64, 95% CI: 0.57–0.71), ischemic stroke (RR = 0.71, 95% CI: 0.62–0.82), and cardiovascular mortality (RR = 0.69, 95% CI: 0.54–0.88),[4] findings that are similar in magnitude to results from prior meta-analyses.[6] Absolute benefits in these trials were greater for those with higher baseline risk of atherosclerotic CVD and were not limited to subgroups with hyperlipidemia. The relative reduction in the risk of cardiovascular outcomes was similar across strata defined by cardiovascular risk score, baseline lipid levels, and presence of diabetes, hypertension, metabolic syndrome, or renal dysfunction.[4]

The RR reduction associated with statin treatment does not appear to vary by race/ethnicity, sex, or age,[4] with the caveat that most primary prevention trials did not include racially/ethnically diverse cohorts or individuals older than 75 years of age and therefore lacked the statistical power to detect small differences in these subpopulations. Men and women appear to experience similar reductions in risk of cardiovascular events and deaths with statins compared with placebo[5]; because women face a lower absolute risk of cardiovascular events, they derive a smaller absolute benefit compared with men.[7] With regard to age, data are not adequate to inform whether statins are sufficiently effective and safe in adults older than 75 years of age.[8] Although older adults have the highest risk of incident atherosclerotic CVD, prior observational studies have suggested that LDL-C levels have a lower magnitude of association with cardiovascular outcomes in older adults, and statin use may be associated with greater side effects in the elderly,[9–11] raising concerns about the balance of benefits and harms in this population.[12]

Although primary prevention trials have evaluated statin medications ranging from low to high doses, most trials have compared a single dose with placebo treatment rather than evaluating dose-escalation strategies, and most have tested moderate-dose statins.[4,6] Direct evidence for decreasing risk of CVD events with increasing statin intensity comes from trials among those with a history of coronary heart disease that were powered to compare different statin intensities across trial arms.[13] Indirect evidence comes from meta-analyses of trials that included patients with and without atherosclerotic CVD showing a consistent relationship between the magnitude of LDL-C lowering and the degree of reduction in major vascular events.[13,14] However, head-to-head comparisons of various statin doses for primary prevention remains a priority area for future research.

Statins Are Safe When Used for Primary Prevention of Atherosclerotic Cardiovascular Disease

A concern related to the lifelong use of statins for primary prevention is the potential for rare adverse events that may not be detectable in randomized trials, which tend to have 5 years of follow-up on average. However, extensive real world experience with statins over the past 2 decades and meta-analyses including tens of thousands of patients enrolled in clinical trials suggest that statins are remarkably safe when used for primary prevention. Concerns about toxicities such as the increased risk of diabetes, myopathy, liver damage, hemorrhagic stroke, and cognitive difficulties have largely not borne out: independently performed meta-analyses of primary prevention trials have shown that patients randomized to statin therapy experience similar rates of adverse events and adverse event-related treatment withdrawal compared with those receiving placebo.[4–6] A recent meta-analysis commissioned by the USPSTF found no association between statin treatment and drug withdrawal due to adverse events (RR = 0.95, 95% CI: 0.7–1.21) or serious adverse events (RR = 0.99; 95% CI: 0.94–1.04).[4] The study found no evidence that statins increase the risk of myalgias (RR = 0.96, 95% CI: 0.79–1.16), elevated liver enzymes (RR = 1.10, 95% CI: 0.90–1.35), or cancer (RR = 1.02, 95% CI: 0.90–1.16).[4] There was also no apparent increased risk of rhabdomyolysis, myopathy, renal dysfunction, or cognitive harms, although few trials evaluated these outcomes and therefore estimates were imprecise.[4]

The possibility that statins may result in a slight increased risk of type 2 diabetes was raised in a meta-analysis of trials from 2010 that included a mix of patients with and without prior CVD (odds ratio = 1.09; 95% CI: 1.02–1.17).[15] Subsequent analyses confirmed this finding and identified a graded relationship between statin intensity and degree of diabetes risk.[16–18] The USPSTF-commissioned meta-analysis limited to primary prevention trials did not find a statistically significant increase in the risk of diabetes in the 6 primary prevention trials that reported on diabetes incidence (RR = 1.05, 95% CI: 0.9–1.20).[4] However, the JUPITER trial, which evaluated rosuvastatin compared with placebo in subjects without a history of CVD, identified an increased risk of diabetes among those receiving rosuvastatin (RR = 1.25; 95% CI: 1.05–1.49). This increased incidence of diabetes was concentrated among patients with a higher baseline risk for diabetes.[19]

Summary of Recommendations from the American College of Cardiology/American Heart Association and the US Preventive Services Task Force

On balance, the accumulated evidence indicates that the benefits gained from preventing incident CVD events and deaths outweigh the harms associated with the rare occurrence of side effects related to the use of statins for primary prevention. With several primary prevention trials demonstrating effectiveness among patients enrolled based on CVD risk factors without requirements for elevated cholesterol levels, recent recommendations have moved away from defining target treatment populations based only on explicit LDL-C thresholds[20] and toward targeting patients more broadly based on estimated risk of atherosclerotic CVD.[2,3,21–23] Differences among the various guidelines reflect current gaps in research evidence.[24]

The 2013 ACC/AHA guidelines[3] and the 2016 USPSTF recommendations[2] both use the Pooled Cohort Equations calculator to calculate 10-year risk.[3] The ACC/AHA guidelines recommend treating with moderate- or high-intensity statins, compared with low- or moderate-dose statins generally recommended by the USPSTF. Among patients aged 40 to 75 years with diabetes, an LDL-C level between 71 and 189 mg/dL, and no clinical atherosclerotic disease, ACC/AHA guidelines recommend initiating statin therapy: high-intensity for those with a 10-year calculated risk of ≥7.5% and moderate-intensity for others. In contrast, USPTF recommendations do not recommend treating patients with diabetes who have a calculated 10-year risk of less than 7.5%.

A major critique of these risk-based guidelines is that they expand indications for statin therapy to a much larger population compared with prior guidelines that were based on target LDL-C levels. Additional concerns have included the costs associated with treating more individuals over a long timeframe and a reliance on pharmacotherapy that fails to fully acknowledge the role of lifestyle modifications. Both sets of guidelines acknowledge the scarcity of data to inform primary prevention among persons older than 75 years of age, suggesting decisions should be individualized based on clinical judgment and patient preference.[2,3] Despite the paucity of effectiveness and safety data among the elderly, the absolute benefit of statin therapy is proportionate to the absolute risk of CVD events, which increases with age. However, this clinical advantage may be offset from a small increase in rates of adverse events.[12]

Statins Are Cost-Effective When Used for Primary Prevention

Cost-effectiveness evaluations compare the incremental costs and incremental benefits of an intervention with the status quo and evaluate whether the intervention represents a worthwhile investment from a health system perspective.[25] Typically, an incremental cost-effectiveness ratio (ICER) <$50,000 per quality-adjusted life year is considered very cost-effective (or "high value") from the US health system perspective.[26]

The cost-effectiveness of statin therapy for primary prevention depends on the following: (1) cost of statin therapy, currently around $100 for a year's supply of generic statins; (2) savings resulting from cardiac events averted by statin therapy; (3) underlying risk of cardiac events in the population being evaluated (the higher the absolute risk, the greater the clinical benefit and therefore the more cost-effective); and (4) costs and quality-of-life decrements associated with side effects related to statin therapy, particularly the potential risk of diabetes.

Given the declining costs of generic statins, several studies have shown that primary prevention with statins is very cost-effective among populations for whom it is recommended.[12,27,28] For instance, in a microsimulation model of US adults aged 45 to 75 years, Pandya and colleagues[28] showed that using the current 10-year atherosclerotic CVD risk threshold at which statin therapy is recommended by the ACC/AHA (≥7.5% risk of a major cardiovascular event over 10 years) would make statin therapy for primary prevention very cost-effective, with an ICER of $37,000 per quality-adjusted life year.

When individualizing the decision to initiate statin therapy for primary prevention, it should be noted that the effectiveness (and hence cost-effectiveness) of statin therapy is sensitive to patients' willingness to take a daily pill.[27,28] Many patients, such as those with hypertension, may already be taking other medications, so that the addition of a daily statin pill may not affect the patient's overall quality of life. For others, a daily pill may represent a significant "disutility," or decrement in quality of life. The cost-effectiveness of statin therapy for primary prevention is sensitive to this disutility: for the subset of patients for whom the daily statin pill would substantially reduce their perceived quality of life, the therapy may not be cost-effective. Although this may seem self-evident, it highlights the importance of shared decision-making when initiating statin therapy for primary prevention.

CLINICAL MANAGEMENT FOR USE OF STATINS FOR PRIMARY PREVENTION IN PATIENTS WITHOUT ATHEROSCLEROTIC CARDIOVASCULAR DISEASE
Statins Are Underutilized for Primary Prevention

Despite the extensive clinical evidence of effectiveness of statins in primary prevention, real-world utilization of statin therapy among persons without CVD remains low. In a cohort study using the Medical Expenditure Panel Survey, investigators noted that although statin use in the community is increasing, fewer than half of all individuals with dyslipidemia who did not have preexisting CVD or diabetes were using statins in 2012 to 2013.[29] Three subgroups had lower-than-average use of statins: women, racial/ethnic minorities, and the uninsured. Another study using a large national registry of patients in all 50 states found that statins were prescribed in only 32%, 47%, and 61% of patients with severe dyslipidemia in the age groups 30 to 39 years, 40 to 49 years, and 50 to 59 years, respectively.[30] These studies demonstrate a large evidence-practice gap in statin therapy for primary prevention, representing a substantial opportunity for improving the cardiovascular health of the population.

Disparate Clinical Guidelines and Implications for Clinical Practice
Initiating statin therapy
Although the AHA/ACC guidelines and the USPSTF recommendations use a similar approach to determining eligibility for statin therapy, differences can complicate the clinical decision on initiating statins for primary prevention.[2,3,21–23] The authors' approach is outlined in later discussion.

First, the authors identify patients with clinical atherosclerotic CVD (acute coronary syndromes, or a history of myocardial infarction, stable or unstable angina, coronary or other arterial revascularization, stroke, transient ischemic attack, or peripheral arterial disease presumed to be of atherosclerotic origin). This group is a very high-risk group that is eligible for high-intensity statin therapy for secondary prevention.

Second, the authors identify patients with severe dyslipidemia (eg, LDL-C ≥190 mg/dL) with or without a family history of premature CVD. These patients should be considered for high-intensity statin therapy. Note that some of these highest-risk individuals may benefit from combination lipid-lowering therapy, which is beyond the scope of this article.[31]

Third, the authors stratify patients with diabetes who are 40 to 75 years old, without clinical atherosclerotic CVD, and have an LDL-C between 71 and 189 mg/dL. In this subgroup, they consider starting a high-intensity statin if the 10-year estimated CVD risk is ≥7.5%, and a moderate-intensity statin among others.

Fourth, for individuals who do not meet the above criteria, the authors estimate the patient's 10-year risk of major cardiovascular events using a calculator based on the Pooled Cohort Equations.[32] Although imperfect, this calculator is the only US-based CVD risk prediction tool that has been externally validated in other US-based populations. These tools can be accessed using an online calculator (http://tools.acc.org/ASCVD-Risk-estimator/) or medical calculator apps.

Fifth, for individuals aged 40 to 75 years without preexisting CVD with a 10-year risk score of ≥10%, the authors consider initiating at least a moderate-intensity statin. The AHA/ACC guidelines recommend treating with a moderate- to high-potency statin, and considerations such as degree of risk may determine the choice of high-intensity statin in this group.

Sixth, for individuals aged 40 to 75 years without preexisting CVD, at least one CVD risk factor (hypertension, smoking, or dyslipidemia), and a 10-year risk score of ≥7.5% but less than 10%, the authors would consider moderate-intensity statin therapy (in this subgroup of patients, ACC/AHA would recommend moderate- to high-intensity statin therapy; USPSTF recommends low- to moderate-intensity statin therapy).

Finally, the authors carefully weigh the risks and benefits of statin therapy in patients for whom the evidence base is relatively sparse. Although shared decision-making around the initiation or continuation of statin therapy is important for all patients, it is particularly so in groups such as the elderly, for whom the evidence base is weak. The authors therefore strongly recommend that discussions with older adults incorporate considerations of uncertain, potentially larger clinical benefit, patient preference regarding preventive medications, and overall competing risks from other comorbidities. The use of visual tools for shared decision-making (eg, https://statindecisionaid.mayoclinic.org/) may improve the quality of the conversation by facilitating effective communication of benefit and risk.

Choosing the intensity of statin therapy for primary prevention

Starting with low- or moderate-intensity statin therapy may be appropriate in individuals at higher-than-average risk of statin-related complications. Individuals at higher risk include those with impaired renal or hepatic function, those receiving concomitant medications that affect statin metabolism, and those with a history of hemorrhagic stroke.[3] Persons of Asian ancestry require lower doses of statins to achieve similar LDL-C reductions as do Caucasian populations, so that lower starting doses may be appropriate.[3,33] A maximum dose of 40 mg is recommended among individuals receiving simvastatin, because the 80-mg dose is associated with an increased risk of rhabdomyolysis.[34,35] A final consideration may be that most health care plans offer tiered cost sharing: generic statins typically have substantially lower out-of-pocket costs than brand-name statins and cost may be related to adherence in some patients.[36]

Monitoring statin therapy

The ACC/AHA guidelines recommend checking alanine transaminase (ALT) levels at baseline and starting a low-dose statin if baseline ALT is ≥3 times the upper limit of normal.[3] If baseline transaminase levels are normal, no additional monitoring is recommended. Although a baseline lipid profile is required to estimate risk based on Pooled Cohort Equations, the role of follow-up lipid panels is questionable because both the ACC/AHA and the USPSTF guidelines have moved away from targeting specific LDL-C levels. Measuring creatinine kinase at baseline is not recommended, but may be useful in individuals at high risk of myopathy.

A patient report of severe unexplained muscle symptoms after the initiation of statin therapy should prompt discontinuation of the statin followed by an evaluation for rhabdomyolysis, an extremely rare event, occurring in less than 1 per 10,000 individuals treated for 5 years.[5] Most commonly, mild to moderate symptoms resolve with temporary discontinuation of statin therapy; in these cases, rechallenge with the same statin at the same dose (to establish causality) or a lower dose or alternative statin is appropriate. Before giving up on statin therapy or labeling an individual as being "statin intolerant," clinicians should note that most patients who initially report muscle complaints with statin therapy are eventually able to tolerate the original or an alternative statin.[37,38]

Statins are contraindicated in women who are pregnant or nursing. Statins use in women of childbearing potential should include emphasis on the need for effective contraception. Patients receiving multiple additional medications that could interact with statins may need close follow-up, including individuals older than 75 years of age, those who have undergone solid organ transplantation, or persons receiving antiretroviral therapies for HIV.

The Importance of Discussing Lifestyle Modifications

Some have suggested that focusing on statin pharmacotherapy for primary prevention is misplaced, and more emphasis should be given to lifestyle modification that is known to play a role in reducing CVD risk. Focusing on lifestyle modification in all individuals and recommending statins in those at increased risk for atherosclerotic CVD should not be considered mutually exclusive choices. Clinicians should discuss lifestyle modification before statin therapy and throughout the course of treatment, particularly with each dose escalation or addition of a new lipid-lowering medication. Recommendations[39] include maintaining a normal body weight and consuming a dietary pattern that emphasizes intake of vegetables, fruits, and whole grains and limits intake of sweets, sugar-sweetened beverages, and red meats; engaging in regular aerobic physical activity (moderate-grade evidence suggests reductions in LDL-C 3.0–6.0 mg/dL and systolic blood pressure by 2-5 mm Hg)[39]; and refraining from smoking tobacco.

AREAS OF UNCERTAINTY

As noted above, adults older than 75 were underrepresented in the randomized trials, resulting in uncertainty about the efficacy and safety of statins for primary prevention in older populations. If statins are assumed to be as effective in older adults as they were in the populations enrolled in the randomized clinical trials, statins would be cost-effective for primary prevention in this population.[12] However, even a small increase in geriatric-specific adverse effects could offset the cardiovascular benefit,[12] necessitating a careful and individualized consideration of benefits and risk.

Persons with chronic kidney disease are at an increased risk of coronary heart disease.[40] However, the relative reduction in major vascular events with statin therapy may be smaller in patients with lower estimated glomerular filtration rates.[41] Thus, patients with chronic kidney disease and not receiving dialysis may need larger doses of statins compared with individuals with normal kidney function to achieve equivalent risk reductions, although the small increase in risk of adverse events calls for close follow-up during dose escalation. Patients receiving dialysis for end-stage renal disease appeared to derive no statistically significant benefit from statin therapy.[41]

Similarly, persons living with HIV appear to be at an increased risk of atherosclerotic CVD,[42,43] likely related to chronic inflammation, adverse effects of antiretroviral therapies, or increased prevalence of nontraditional risk factors, such as chronic stress or stimulant drug use. It is unclear whether statins improve clinical outcomes among persons living with HIV who do not have preexisting CVD. Pending results of ongoing studies, the authors' approach to statin therapy for primary prevention among persons living with HIV is as follows. They use a similar approach to deciding eligibility for statin therapy among persons living with controlled HIV infection as they would in the general population, estimating risk using the Pooled Cohort Equations (which have been shown to have reasonable discrimination among HIV-infected cohorts).[44] If the decision is made to start statin therapy, the authors choose a statin that has minimal interactions with antiretroviral therapies and start with a low dose: atorvastatin 10 mg, except for patients receiving ritonavir-based protease inhibitor therapies, for whom the authors prefer pitavastatin. Rosuvastatin and pravastatin are reasonable alternatives in this population, whereas simvastatin and lovastatin are not given the risk of drug interactions with commonly prescribed antiretroviral therapies. The authors clinically monitor patients for symptoms of hepatotoxicity or myopathy.

Finally, given the central role of the Pooled Cohort Equations in determining eligibility for statin therapy, it is important to be cognizant of their limitations.[32] There are some concerns that these equations may overestimate risks for atherosclerotic CVD, particularly at the lower end of the risk spectrum. They do not consider novel risk markers such as coronary calcium and serum CRP, which may help further stratify risk (see Mark J. Pletcher and Andrew E. Moran's article, "Cardiovascular Risk Assessment," in this issue for further details). Although white and African American populations are included in the cohorts used to derive these equations, there is uncertainty regarding risk assessment for other racial and ethnic groups; these equations may underestimate risk in South Asian Americans and overestimate risk in East-Asian Americans and Hispanics.

SUMMARY

The weight of high-quality evidence argues in favor of using statin therapy for primary prevention of CVD among individuals who meet eligibility criteria proposed by the ACC/AHA or the USPSTF. Clinicians should take the time to explain the benefits and risks in terms patients are likely to understand and to carefully elicit patient preferences regarding receiving a daily pill for primary prevention. Online or app-based calculators and shared decision-making tools may facilitate effective communication around this important decision. Statin therapy is a cost-effective but underutilized approach to primary prevention of atherosclerotic CVD.

REFERENCES

1. Mozaffarian D, Benjamin EJ, Go AS, et al. Heart Disease and Stroke Statistics-2016 Update: a report from the American Heart Association. Circulation 2016; 133(4):e38–360.

2. Bibbins-Domingo K, Grossman DC, Curry SJ, et al. Statin use for the primary prevention of cardiovascular disease in adults: US Preventive Services Task Force Recommendation Statement. JAMA 2016;316(19):1997–2007.

3. Stone NJ, Robinson JG, Lichtenstein AH, et al. 2013 ACC/AHA guideline on the treatment of blood cholesterol to reduce atherosclerotic cardiovascular risk in adults: a report of the American College of Cardiology/American Heart Association Task Force on Practice Guidelines. Circulation 2014;129(25 Suppl 2):S1–45.

4. Chou R, Dana T, Blazina I, et al. Statins for prevention of cardiovascular disease in adults: evidence report and systematic review for the US Preventive Services Task Force. JAMA 2016;316(19):2008–24.

5. Fulcher J, O'Connell R, Voysey M, et al. Efficacy and safety of LDL-lowering therapy among men and women: meta-analysis of individual data from 174,000 participants in 27 randomised trials. Lancet 2015;385(9976):1397–405.

6. Taylor F, Huffman MD, Macedo AF, et al. Statins for the primary prevention of cardiovascular disease. Cochrane Database Syst Rev 2013;(1):CD004816.

7. Mosca L. Sex, statins, and statistics. Lancet 2015;385(9976):1368–9.

8. Sever PS, Dahlof B, Poulter NR, et al. Prevention of coronary and stroke events with atorvastatin in hypertensive patients who have average or lower-than-average cholesterol concentrations, in the Anglo-Scandinavian Cardiac Outcomes Trial–Lipid Lowering Arm (ASCOT-LLA): a multicentre randomised controlled trial. Lancet 2003;361(9364):1149–58.

9. Kronmal RA, Cain KC, Ye Z, et al. Total serum cholesterol levels and mortality risk as a function of age. A report based on the Framingham data. Arch Intern Med 1993;153(9):1065–73.

10. Krumholz HM, Seeman TE, Merrill SS, et al. Lack of association between cholesterol and coronary heart disease mortality and morbidity and all-cause mortality in persons older than 70 years. JAMA 1994;272(17):1335–40.

11. Schiattarella GG, Perrino C, Magliulo F, et al. Statins and the elderly: recent evidence and current indications. Aging Clin Exp Res 2012;24(3 Suppl):47–55.

12. Odden MC, Pletcher MJ, Coxson PG, et al. Cost-effectiveness and population impact of statins for primary prevention in adults aged 75 years or older in the United States. Ann Intern Med 2015;162(8):533–41.

13. Mihaylova B, Emberson J, Blackwell L, et al. The effects of lowering LDL cholesterol with statin therapy in people at low risk of vascular disease: meta-analysis of individual data from 27 randomised trials. Lancet 2012;380(9841):581–90.

14. Silverman MG, Ference BA, Im K, et al. Association between lowering LDL-C and cardiovascular risk reduction among different therapeutic interventions: a systematic review and meta-analysis. JAMA 2016;316(12):1289–97.

15. Sattar N, Preiss D, Murray HM, et al. Statins and risk of incident diabetes: a collaborative meta-analysis of randomised statin trials. Lancet 2010;375(9716): 735–42.

16. Preiss D, Seshasai SR, Welsh P, et al. Risk of incident diabetes with intensive-dose compared with moderate-dose statin therapy: a meta-analysis. JAMA 2011;305(24):2556–64.

17. Wang S, Cai R, Yuan Y, et al. Association between reductions in low-density lipoprotein cholesterol with statin therapy and the risk of new-onset diabetes: a meta-analysis. Sci Rep 2017;7:39982.

18. Mills EJ, Wu P, Chong G, et al. Efficacy and safety of statin treatment for cardiovascular disease: a network meta-analysis of 170,255 patients from 76 randomized trials. QJM 2011;104(2):109–24.

19. Ridker PM, Danielson E, Fonseca FA, et al. Rosuvastatin to prevent vascular events in men and women with elevated C-reactive protein. N Engl J Med 2008;359(21):2195–207.

20. National Cholesterol Education Program (NCEP) Expert Panel on Detection, Evaluation, and Treatment of High Blood Cholesterol in Adults (Adult Treatment Panel III). Third report of the National Cholesterol Education Program (NCEP) expert panel on detection, evaluation, and treatment of high blood cholesterol in adults (Adult Treatment Panel III) final report. Circulation 2002;106(25):3143–421.

21. Anderson TJ, Gregoire J, Hegele RA, et al. 2012 update of the Canadian Cardiovascular Society guidelines for the diagnosis and treatment of dyslipidemia for the prevention of cardiovascular disease in the adult. Can J Cardiol 2013; 29(2):151–67.

22. Catapano AL, Graham I, De Backer G, et al. 2016 ESC/EAS Guidelines for the Management of Dyslipidaemias: the Task Force for the Management of Dyslipidaemias of the European Society of Cardiology (ESC) and European Atherosclerosis Society (EAS) developed with the special contribution of the European Association for Cardiovascular Prevention & Rehabilitation (EACPR). Atherosclerosis 2016;253:281–344.

23. JBS3 Board. Joint British Societies' consensus recommendations for the prevention of cardiovascular disease (JBS3). Heart 2014;100(Suppl 2):ii1–67.

24. Greenland P, Bonow RO. Interpretation and use of another statin guideline. JAMA 2016;316(19):1977–9.

25. Sanders GD, Neumann PJ, Basu A, et al. Recommendations for conduct, methodological practices, and reporting of cost-effectiveness analyses: second panel on cost-effectiveness in health and medicine. JAMA 2016;316(10):1093–103.

26. Anderson JL, Heidenreich PA, Barnett PG, et al. ACC/AHA statement on cost/value methodology in clinical practice guidelines and performance measures: a report of the American College of Cardiology/American Heart Association Task Force on Performance Measures and Task Force on Practice Guidelines. Circulation 2014;129(22):2329–45.

27. Lazar LD, Pletcher MJ, Coxson PG, et al. Cost-effectiveness of statin therapy for primary prevention in a low-cost statin era. Circulation 2011;124(2):146–53.

28. Pandya A, Sy S, Cho S, et al. Cost-effectiveness of 10-year risk thresholds for initiation of statin therapy for primary prevention of cardiovascular disease. JAMA 2015;314(2):142–50.

29. Salami JA, Warraich H, Valero-Elizondo J, et al. National trends in statin use and expenditures in the US adult population from 2002 to 2013: insights from the Medical Expenditure Panel Survey. JAMA Cardiol 2017;2(1):56–65.

30. Al-Kindi SG, DeCicco A, Longenecker CT, et al. Rate of statin prescription in younger patients with severe dyslipidemia. JAMA Cardiol 2017;2(4):451–2 [Epub ahead of print].

31. Kazi DS, Moran AE, Coxson PG, et al. Cost-effectiveness of PCSK9 inhibitor therapy in patients with heterozygous familial hypercholesterolemia or atherosclerotic cardiovascular disease. JAMA 2016;316(7):743–53.

32. Goff DC Jr, Lloyd-Jones DM, Bennett G, et al. 2013 ACC/AHA guideline on the assessment of cardiovascular risk: a report of the American College of Cardiology/American Heart Association Task Force on Practice Guidelines. Circulation 2014;129(25 Suppl 2):S49–73.

33. Liao JK. Safety and efficacy of statins in Asians. Am J Cardiol 2007;99(3):410–4.

34. de Lemos JA, Blazing MA, Wiviott SD, et al. Early intensive vs a delayed conservative simvastatin strategy in patients with acute coronary syndromes: phase Z of the A to Z trial. JAMA 2004;292(11):1307–16.

35. Armitage J, Bowman L, Wallendszus K, et al. Intensive lowering of LDL cholesterol with 80 mg versus 20 mg simvastatin daily in 12,064 survivors of myocardial infarction: a double-blind randomised trial. Lancet 2010;376(9753):1658–69.

36. Gagne JJ, Choudhry NK, Kesselheim AS, et al. Comparative effectiveness of generic and brand-name statins on patient outcomes: a cohort study. Ann Intern Med 2014;161(6):400–7.

37. Mampuya WM, Frid D, Rocco M, et al. Treatment strategies in patients with statin intolerance: the Cleveland Clinic experience. Am Heart J 2013;166(3):597–603.

38. Zhang H, Plutzky J, Skentzos S, et al. Discontinuation of statins in routine care settings: a cohort study. Ann Intern Med 2013;158(7):526–34.

39. Eckel RH, Jakicic JM, Ard JD, et al. 2013 AHA/ACC guideline on lifestyle management to reduce cardiovascular risk: a report of the American College of Cardiology/American Heart Association Task Force on Practice Guidelines. J Am Coll Cardiol 2014;63(25 Pt B):2960–84.

40. Go AS, Chertow GM, Fan D, et al. Chronic kidney disease and the risks of death, cardiovascular events, and hospitalization. N Engl J Med 2004;351(13):1296–305.

41. Herrington WG, Emberson J, Mihaylova B, et al. Impact of renal function on the effects of LDL cholesterol lowering with statin-based regimens: a meta-analysis of individual participant data from 28 randomised trials. Lancet Diabetes Endocrinol 2016;4(10):829–39.

42. Freiberg MS, Chang CC, Kuller LH, et al. HIV infection and the risk of acute myocardial infarction. JAMA Intern Med 2013;173(8):614–22.

43. U.S. National Institutes of Health. Evaluating the Use of Pivastatin to Reduce the Risk of Cardiovascular Disease in HIV-Infected Adults (REPRIEVE). 2015. Available at: https://clinicaltrials.gov/ct2/show/NCT02344290?term=REPRIEVE+HIV&rank=1. Accessed February 22, 2017.

44. Feinstein MJ, Nance RM, Drozd DR, et al. Assessing and refining myocardial infarction risk estimation among patients with human immunodeficiency virus: a study by the Centers for AIDS Research Network of Integrated Clinical Systems. JAMA Cardiol 2017;2(2):155–62.

Screening for Hypertension and Lowering Blood Pressure for Prevention of Cardiovascular Disease Events

Anthony J. Viera, MD, MPH

KEYWORDS

- Hypertension • High blood pressure • Screening
- Cardiovascular disease prevention • Ambulatory blood pressure monitoring

KEY POINTS

- High blood pressure (BP) is the single greatest contributor to the global burden of disease.
- BP-lowering therapy reduces risk of stroke about 35%, myocardial infarction about 25%, and heart failure by more than 50%.
- Ambulatory BP monitoring is recommended to confirm the diagnosis of hypertension in most patients before initiating drug therapy; home BP monitoring is an alternative.
- Treatment guidelines are stratified by age (<60 vs >60 years) and include cutoffs for recommended treatment BPs and target BP goals.
- Quality improvement efforts for BP control include incorporation of registries, evidence-based treatment algorithms with specialized titration visits, and regular reporting of control rates.

THE IMPORTANCE OF HYPERTENSION

Increased blood pressure (BP) is the strongest modifiable risk factor for cardiovascular disease (CVD) and the most important contributor to global mortality, contributing to an estimated 9.4 million deaths per year.[1] CVD morbidity and mortality are correlated positively with the degree of elevation of BP, without any evidence of a threshold down to at least 115/75 mm Hg.[2] For every increase of 20 mm Hg in the systolic BP above 115 mm Hg, the CVD risk doubles.[2]

Disclosure Statement: Dr A.J. Viera has no disclosures.
Department of Family Medicine, University of North Carolina at Chapel Hill, 590 Manning Drive, CB 7595, Chapel Hill, NC 27599, USA
E-mail address: viera@med.unc.edu

Med Clin N Am 101 (2017) 701–712
http://dx.doi.org/10.1016/j.mcna.2017.03.003
0025-7125/17/© 2017 Elsevier Inc. All rights reserved.

The goal of a population strategy to reduce CVD events attributable to elevated BP is to reduce average BP such that the distribution curve "shifts to the left." Population-level interventions could include policies that reduce sodium consumption (eg, content of prepackaged foods).[3] The conventional clinical approach to reduce CVD events attributable to elevated BP relies on identifying people above an arbitrary threshold or cutpoint, who are "diagnosed" as having hypertension. Predominant guidelines currently recommend a threshold of 140 mm Hg systolic (150 mm Hg for older adults) or 90 mm Hg diastolic based on office BP measurements.[4–6] At this level of BP, clinical intervention (labeling, evaluating, treating with medications) offers net benefit, that is, the weight of the evidence suggests that it does more good than harm. Because hypertension is an asymptomatic condition, the clinical strategy relies on screening to identify people for whom risk-reducing strategies can be offered.

EPIDEMIOLOGY OF HYPERTENSION

Hypertension affects 1 in 3 American adults over the age of 18, making it the most commonly seen condition in adult primary care practices.[7,8] Its high prevalence along with average longer life expectancy translate into substantial population exposure to this risk factor. Prevalence increases with age such that approximately 7% of 20- to 34-year-olds are affected, that 54% of 55- to 64-year-olds have high BP, and that, among those 75 years and older in the United States, nearly 80% have hypertension.[8]

Men and women between the ages of 55 and 64 are approximately equally likely to have high BP, with nearly 54% of the population affected (**Table 1**).[8] Before this age, men are more commonly affected, and after these ages more females are affected. Black women most commonly have hypertension (43%), with black men following (42%).[8] Approximately 30% of white men have high BP, whereas 28% of white women are affected.[8] About 27% of Mexican American men and women have hypertension.[8] People who are normotensive at 55 years of age still have a 90% life-time risk for developing hypertension.[9]

Fortunately, treatment of hypertension with BP-lowering medications reduces the risk of heart failure, stroke, myocardial infarction, chronic kidney disease, and cognitive decline. Left untreated, hypertension may lead to vascular and renal damage, which with time could become treatment resistant.[5] The percentage of people who know they have hypertension, who are treated, and who have controlled BP has increased. From 2005 to 2010, nearly 82% of adults with hypertension were aware

Table 1 Prevalence of hypertension by age and sex categories		
Sex	Age Group (y)	Prevalence (%)
Male	20–34	8.6
	35–44	22.6
	45–54	36.8
	55–64	54.6
	65–74	62.0
	≥75	76.4
Female	20–34	6.2
	35–44	18.3
	45–54	32.7
	55–64	53.7
	65–74	67.8
	≥75	79.9

of their status (up from 75% in prior years), and approximately 75% were taking medication. Nearly 53% of these patients had controlled BP.[8] Of the myriad of preventive services clinicians can offer, BP-lowering treatment is one of the most beneficial. Among the US population, each 10% increase in the number of people with controlled BP would prevent 14,000 premature deaths.[10]

REDUCING CARDIOVASCULAR EVENTS

In a metaanalysis of clinical trials, antihypertensive therapy has been shown to reduce stroke by about 35% to 40%, myocardial infarction by 20% to 25%, and heart failure by more than 50%.[11] These data support the importance of treating patients to reduce BP and, more important, to prevent the morbidity and mortality associated with hypertension; notably, these effects are highly generalizable and broadly comparable across diverse populations.[11]

The antihypertensive clinical trials have either enrolled patients with established CVD or who had increased CVD risk or higher levels of BP. It is unlikely that a placebo-controlled trial evaluating the treatment of mild hypertension will ever be done, given the large number of patients who would need to be followed for many years to accrue enough events to make inferences about mortality benefit. Although there have been no trials the examining primary prevention of CVD events among patients exclusively with mild hypertension, the weight of the evidence supports a treatment benefit.[12] Several of the secondary prevention trials even show benefits among the nonhypertensive participant subgroups.

TECHNIQUES FOR MEASURING BLOOD PRESSURE
Office Blood Pressure Measurement

Because mercury instruments have been eliminated from clinical settings, measurement of BP in the office using either aneroid sphygmomanometer or an automatic oscillometric monitor is the most commonly used technique to assess BP. Automatic oscillometric devices estimate systolic and diastolic BP based on a pressure waveform, and particular algorithms vary based on manufacturer. A list of validated devices is maintained at www.dableducational.org. Regardless of method, accurate measurement of office BP is challenging, particularly in busy practices, where BP is often measured by medical assistants or nurses as part of the vital signs before the patient is seen by the clinician. Proper technique (**Table 2**) is important but may not be followed routinely.[13]

The proper technique for measurement of BP requires a patient to have had at least a 5-minute sitting period followed by correct application of the appropriate sized cuff on the bare upper arm.[13] The patient is to be seated upright with his or her feet flat on

Table 2 Common technical errors in office blood pressure measurement	
Technical Problem	**Estimated Degree of Error, mm Hg Systolic/Diastolic[15]**
Arm not supported	1–7/5–11
Back unsupported	6–10
Cuff size incorrect	−8 to +10/2–8
Failure to allow sufficient rest	Variable
Faulty equipment	Variable
Talking during measurement	7/8

the floor and avoid talking or moving. The arm is to rest on a flat surface at heart level. Then the measurement is taken and recorded. When using the auscultatory method, the manometer should be placed at eye level, and the room should be quiet enough for the observer to hear the Korotkoff sounds.[13,14]

Observers introduce measurement error in several ways. Some are related to the procedure itself: improper cuff selection, positioning, or application; too rapid deflation of the cuff; or incorrect Korotkoff sound used.[15] Others are related to bias, a common one being terminal digit bias, or the tendency to over-record '0' or '5' as the terminal digit in an auscultatory-based measurement. Automatic BP devices are increasing in use in office practices. Such devices eliminate some of the observer factors, such as speed of cuff deflation, variability in Korotkoff sound interpretation, and terminal digit bias, but still depend on accurate cuff size and placement, and proper patient preparation and positioning.

Even when measurement of BP is performed with no technical errors and the measurement is accurate, a single BP reading may not represent a person's usual BP because of the many factors, both inherent and external, that influence variability of BP. For example, a full bladder may raise the BP by 15/10 mm Hg.[15] Therefore, a person's BP is not generally judged by a single office reading. Instead, a combination of repeat same-visit measurements and follow-up visit measurements are recommended.

Ambulatory Blood Pressure Monitoring

With ambulatory BP monitoring (ABPM), the patient wears a monitor during most of his or her usual activities for a defined period, typically of 24 hours. The monitor is pre-programmed to take BP measurements at specified intervals, such as every 30 minutes, or every 20 minutes during the awake hours and every 45 minutes during sleep. This type of monitoring provides many individual BP readings that can then be averaged to provide an assessment of the patient's "usual" BP.[16] Measurements can also be grouped into time windows (eg, mean daytime and nighttime BPs).

Automated Office Blood Pressure Measurement

Automated office BP measurement uses a device that is preprogrammed to record several BP measurements in short succession (eg, 1 minute intervals) without an observer present. Devices currently available for incorporating this technique include the BpTRU, Microlife WatchBP Office (Welch Allyn PRO BP 2400), and Omron HEM-907. Automated office BP assessment typically requires between 4 and 7 minutes to obtain a mean BP reading. An advantage of automated office BP is mitigation or elimination of the white coat effect.[17] It is worth noting that the 2016 Canadian Hypertension Education Program recommends automated office BP as the preferred method for office BP measurement.[18]

Home Blood Pressure Monitoring

Home BP monitoring also allows several out-of-office BP measurements to be taken. As such, it can also provide a closer estimate of a person's "true" BP.[19,20] Unlike with ABPM, however, this method relies on the patient to perform the measurements, usually using an automatic oscillometric device on the upper arm. The currently available monitors are relatively reliable and accurate.[19] Many have undergone independent validation studies using standard international protocols. Modern home BP monitors are also easy to use, requiring only wrapping the cuff around the arm and pushing a button. Many monitors have a memory so that readings are stored and can be reviewed at a later date (eliminating reliance on self-reported written records).

Home BP measurements are generally taken in the morning and in the evening. The readings tend to be more stable than those taken using ABPM, a finding presumed to arise from the fact that the conditions in which they are taken are less variable.[21] Using a minimum number of 5 days of duplicate sets of measurements, it has been shown that a reliable estimate of a patient's usual BP that correlates with 24-hour ABPM (r = 0.70) can be obtained.[22] Although home BP monitoring relies more on patient performance and requires a longer period of use than does ABPM, it is more widely available and less expensive. A list if validated home BP devices is also maintained at the www.dableducational.org website.

SCREENING RECOMMENDATIONS

The most recent US Preventive Services Task Force recommendation regarding hypertension was released October 2015.[23] The task force affirmed its previous "grade A" recommendation to screen all adults over 18 years of age for hypertension.[24] The updated guideline includes a recommendation for screening intervals. The US Preventive Services Task Force recommends annual screening for adults 40 years and older and those at increased risk for high BP. Persons deemed at increased risk include those who have high-normal BP (130–139/85–89 mm Hg), are overweight or obese, or are African American. Adults ages 18 to 39 years with normal BP (<130/85 mm Hg) who do not have other risk factors should be rescreened every 3 to 5 years.[23,25]

In a patient with a single greatly elevated BP reading in the office setting who already has hypertensive-related target organ damage (eg, left ventricular hypertrophy), the diagnosis of hypertension may be made without follow-up readings. For most other patients, the diagnosis of hypertension should be based on at least 2 separately recorded elevated BP recordings. The finding of an elevated BP at an initial should be confirmed at a follow-up visit, preferably with at least 2 BP recordings separated by at least 1 minute each time.[26]

Ideally, for patients for whom the need for BP-lowering therapy is not obvious, ABPM should be used to confirm the diagnosis of hypertension.[5,23] This recommendation was based on a systematic review in which diagnostic and predictive accuracy of different BP methods were evaluated.[25] Office BP measurement thresholds are noted to have poor overall sensitivity and specificity for diagnosing hypertension (**Fig. 1**).[25]

Importantly, several studies have shown that ABPM is superior to office BP in predicting CVD events and mortality.[27–32] One study prospectively followed 1187 subjects with essential hypertension and 205 healthy normotensive control subjects for up to 7.5 years (mean, 3.2) who had baseline off-therapy 24-hour ABPM.[28] The number of combined fatal and nonfatal cardiovascular events per 100 patient-years was 0.47 in the sustained normotension group, 0.49 in the white coat hypertension (elevated office with normal ambulatory BP) group, 1.79 in those with daytime ambulatory hypertension, and 4.99 in those with 24-hour ambulatory hypertension. After adjustment for traditional risk markers for CVD, morbidity did not differ between the normotensive and white coat hypertension groups (P = .83). Compared with the white coat hypertension group, cardiovascular morbidity increased in those with daytime ambulatory hypertension (relative risk, 3.70; 95% confidence interval [CI], 1.13–12.5), with a further increase of morbidity in those with 24-hour ambulatory hypertension (relative risk, 6.26; 95% CI, 1.92–20.32).

In a substudy to the Syst-Eur Trial (Systolic Hypertension in Europe), 808 participants' baseline office BPs (mean of 6 readings) were compared with their 24-hour ambulatory BPs.[31] After a median follow-up of 4.4 years (range 1–110 months), and

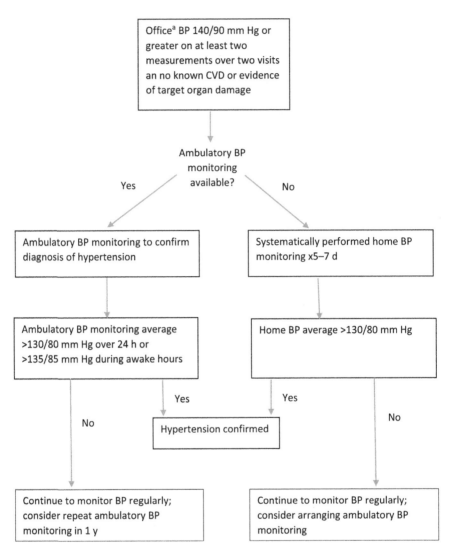

Fig. 1. Approach to screening and diagnosis of hypertension. [a] If automated office blood pressure (BP) is used, out-of-office measurements may not be necessary. CVD, cardiovascular disease.

adjustment for sex, age, previous cardiovascular complications, smoking, and place of residence, a 10-mm Hg higher office systolic BP at baseline was not associated with a worse prognosis, whereas a 10-mm Hg higher 24-hour ambulatory BP was associated with an increased relative hazard rate of most outcome measures (eg, hazard rate, 1.23 [95% CI, 1.00–1.50] for total mortality and 1.34 [95% CI, 1.03–1.75] for cardiovascular mortality). In one of the largest studies comparing office BP and ABPM, baseline office and ambulatory BPs of 5292 initially untreated (or off treatment) hypertensive patients were measured and followed over a median time of 8.4 years.[32] There were 646 deaths, 389 of which were deemed cardiovascular. After adjustment for sex, age, risk indices, and office BP, higher mean values of ambulatory BP were independent predictors for cardiovascular mortality. The relative hazard ratio for each 10-mm Hg increase in daytime systolic BP was 1.12 (95% CI, 1.06–1.18).

A systematic review and cost-effectiveness study formed the basis for the UK's 2011 recommendation to use ABPM to confirm the diagnosis of hypertension.[33,34] The use of ABPM permits recognition of white coat hypertension, which the preponderance of the evidence suggests does not require BP-lowering treatment.[35] Eliminating the misdiagnosis of patients with white coat hypertension as having "true" (or sustained) hypertension saves a large proportion of patients from unnecessary medication. The cost-effectiveness study, which used a Markov model to simulate a hypothetical population of adults 40 years and older, calculated ABPM to be the most cost-effective strategy for the diagnosis of hypertension.[34] It was deemed cost-saving for all groups and resulted in more quality-adjusted life-years for men and women older than 50 years.[34]

Although the task force notes ABPM to be the preferred method for out-of-office BP measurements to use to confirm the diagnosis of hypertension, the guidelines state that home BP monitoring may be an acceptable alternative.[23]

TREATMENT GOALS
Joint National Committee 8 Recommendations

The most recent US guideline on hypertension treatment is the report issued by the panel members appointed to the Joint National Committee 8.[36] Based on a careful review of the evidence available at the time, the guideline issued a grade A recommendation that in the general population aged 60 years or older, pharmacologic treatment (**Fig. 2**) should be initiated to lower BP at a systolic BP of 150 mm Hg or greater or a diastolic BP of 90 mm Hg or greater, and treat to a goal systolic BP of less than 150 mm Hg and goal diastolic BP of less than 90 mm Hg. For patients less than 60 years of age, expert opinion recommendation is to initiate treatment with a systolic BP of 140 mm Hg or greater and treat to a goal of less than 140 mm Hg, and grade A recommendation is a to initiate pharmacologic treatment to lower BP at a diastolic BP of 90 mm Hg or greater and treat to a goal of less than 90 mm Hg. In the population aged 18 years or older with diabetes or chronic kidney disease, the guideline recommends to initiate pharmacologic treatment at a systolic BP of 140 mm Hg or greater, or a diastolic BP of 90 mm Hg or greater, and treat to goal BP of less than 140/90 mm Hg.

Lifestyle Recommendations

Several lifestyle modifications have been shown to reduce BP and are recommended as part of the management of patients with hypertension. These recommendations include weight loss if overweight, exercise, the Dietary Approaches to Stop Hypertension eating plan, reduced dietary sodium intake, and alcohol reduction.[4,12] Unfortunately, the reality is that many patients are unable to initiate and sustain behavioral change, particularly in unsupportive environments. Additionally, although lifestyle modifications may lower the BP, there is limited evidence that these approaches for managing hypertension actually reduce CVD events.

Targeting Lower Blood Pressure Goals

Since the release of the guideline by the Joint National Committee 8 panel members, the SPRINT trial (Systolic Blood Pressure Intervention Trial) was published.[37] This landmark trial offers further insight into BP treatment goals. SPRINT was a randomized trial including 9361 persons 50 years of age and older with a systolic BP of 130 mm Hg

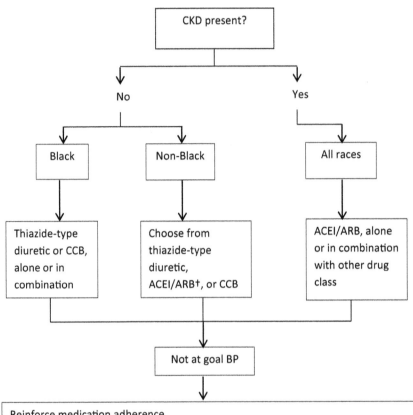

Fig. 2. Drug treatment of hypertension. †, Do not use ACEI and ARB together; ACEI, angiotensin converting enzyme inhibitor; ARB, angiotensin receptor blocker; CCB, calcium channel blocker; CKD, chronic kidney disease.

or greater and either established CVD (20% of the participants) or an increased CVD risk (ie, 61% of participants had a 10-year CVD risk of ≥15%), but without diabetes. The participants were randomized to a systolic BP target of less than 120 mm Hg (intensive treatment) or a target of less than 140 mm Hg (standard treatment). The primary composite outcome was myocardial infarction, other acute coronary syndrome, stroke, heart failure, or death from cardiovascular causes. At baseline, 91% of participants were already on BP-lowering medication(s), and mean BP was 140/78 mm Hg with systolic BP of less than 145 mm Hg in 66%.

At the 1-year follow-up, the mean systolic BP was 136 mm Hg in the standard treatment group and 121 mm Hg in the intensive treatment group. The trial was stopped early after a median follow-up of approximately 3.3 years, when a significantly lower rate of the primary composite outcome was observed in the intensive treatment group compared with the standard treatment group (1.65% vs 2.19% per year; hazard rate, 0.75; 95% CI, 0.64–0.89) All-cause mortality was also 27% lower in the intensive treatment group. Although overall rates of side effects were similar between treatment groups, the rates of serious some adverse events (hypotension, syncope, electrolyte abnormalities, and acute kidney injury) were higher in the intensive treatment group.

The BP measurement method in SPRINT is important to note. Office BP readings were taken using an automated office BP monitor. The automatic monitor was preset to wait 5 minutes before measurement and to automatically take and average 3 consecutive readings without an observer present. As mentioned, such a strategy helps to mitigate the white coat effect.[17] Overall, the SPRINT demonstrated that for a group of nondiabetic patients at increased risk or with established CVD, a lower BP target—when BP is carefully measured—reduces CVD events. However, these findings may not be applicable for a large proportion of individuals with hypertension in primary care. An analysis of the National Health and Nutrition Examination Survey suggests that about 16.7% of people with hypertension would meet SPRINT qualifying criteria.[38] Such patients are more likely to be men of older age, and non-Hispanic whites.

CARDIOVASCULAR DISEASE RISK-BASED APPROACH

As mentioned, the conventional clinical approach in addressing hypertension is to diagnose and offer treatment based on BP level threshold. However, use of a CVD risk-based approach might offer patients a better balance of benefits and risks. For patients at lower levels of BP and lower levels of CVD risk, a CVD risk-based approach can be used to facilitate shared decision-making discussions. Consider a 47-year-old Caucasian woman (nonsmoker) with an office BP of 150/75 mm Hg who has no other risk factors. Using the atherosclerotic cardiovascular disease risk calculator (available at: www.cvriskcalculator.com), she has an estimated 10-year risk of 1% to 2% for heart disease or stroke. Reducing this risk by 20% using BP-lowering medication would confer an absolute risk reduction of only about 0.2%.

With the conventional threshold-based approach, patients with "normal" BP levels may not be offered BP-lowering medications despite having an overall high CVD risk. Consider a 67-year-old man, nonsmoker, with a BP of 138/70 mm Hg, diabetes, and dyslipidemia whose 10-year risk for a CVD event is 40%. BP-lowering medication would offer substantial absolute risk reduction (of about 8%), yet based solely on a BP threshold approach, he would not qualify for treatment.

The modern approach to primary prevention when caring for patients with hypertension should, therefore, consider overall CVD risk. For patients with lower levels of elevated BP or low/intermediate levels of overall CVD risk, shared decision making should be used when considering whether to start or add pharmacologic treatment.

QUALITY OF HYPERTENSION CARE

Despite an array of effective medications and decades of educating the public on the importance of recognizing and treating hypertension, attaining control of BP among patients with hypertension is challenging. According to recent estimates, only 53% of patients with hypertension have their BP under control. Evidence shows that initiation and persistence with medication(s) are far from optimal.[39] Strategies to overcome clinical inertia—the failure of clinicians to intensity therapy—are also needed.[40] In addition to patient factors, there are clinical factors that impede achievement of BP control, such as competing demands and time pressures. Quality improvement strategies for BP control generally include a comprehensive, system-level approach with incorporation of population management principles.[41] For example, at Kaiser-Permanente Northern California, a comprehensive multicomponent quality

---

Box 1
Components of a hypertension population health management strategy

- Develop and disseminate an evidence-based hypertension treatment algorithm in which single-pill combination therapy is considered.
- Use a robust hypertension registry in which patients with hypertension are identified regularly and contacted as needed.
- Provide regular reporting on hypertension control rates.
- Incorporate medical assistant visits 2 to 4 weeks after a medication adjustment to facilitate treatment intensification by primary care clinician.

---

improvement program (**Box 1**) led to a 37% improvement in hypertension control from 2001 to 2009, with more than 80% of hypertension patients having controlled BP.[42]

Implementing comprehensive quality improvement strategies in a nonclosed system can be more challenging, but the principles are similar. Strategies might target not only the system, but also the patients and/or clinicians. For example, engaging patients in self-management using home BP monitoring may improve BP control.[41,43] Auditing clinicians and providing feedback or reminders also may be effective.[41,43] The Health Resources and Services Administration has made available a comprehensive resource for hypertension quality improvement online at: https://www.hrsa.gov/quality/toolbox/measures/hypertension/.

REFERENCES

1. Lim SS, Vos T, Flaxman AD, et al. A comparative risk assessment of burden of disease and injury attributable to 67 risk factors and risk factor clusters in 21 regions, 1990-2010: a systematic analysis for the Global Burden of Disease Study 2010. Lancet 2013;380:2224–60.
2. Lewington S, Clarke R, Qizilbash N, et al, Prospective Studies Collaboration. Age-specific relevance of usual blood pressure to vascular mortality: a meta-analysis of individual data for one million adults in 61 prospective studies. Lancet 2002; 360(9349):1903–13.
3. Coxson PG, Cook NR, Joffres M, et al. Mortality benefits from US population-wide reduction in sodium consumption: projections from 3 modeling approaches. Hypertension 2013;61(3):564–70.
4. Chobanian AV, Barkis GL, Black HR, et al. The seventh report of the Joint National Committee on Prevention, Detection, Evaluation, and Treatment of High Blood Pressure: the JNC 7 report. JAMA 2003;289:2560–72.
5. National Institute for Health and Care Excellence (NICE). Hypertension: clinical management of primary hypertension in adults. August 2011. Available at: https://www.ncbi.nlm.nih.gov/pubmed/22855971. Accessed August, 2011.
6. Weber MA, Schiffrin EL, White WB, et al. Clinical practice guidelines for the management of hypertension in the community a statement by the American Society of Hypertension and the International Society of Hypertension. J Hypertens 2014; 32(1):3–15.
7. Centers for Disease Control and Prevention (CDC). Vital signs: prevalence, treatment, and control of hypertension–United States, 1999–2002 and 2005—2008. MMWR Morb Mortal Wkly Rep 2011;60(04):103–8.
8. Mozaffarian D, Benjamin EJ, Go AS, et al. American Heart Association Statistics committee.; stroke statistics subcommittee. executive summary: heart disease

and stroke statistics–2016 update: a report from the American Heart Association. Circulation 2016;133(4):447–54.

9. Vasan RS, Beiser A, Seshadri S, et al. Residual lifetime risk for developing hypertension in middle-aged women and men: the Framingham Heart Study. JAMA 2002;287:1003–10.

10. Farley TA, Dalal MA, Mostashari F, et al. Deaths preventable in the U.S. by improvements in use of clinical preventive services. Am J Prev Med 2010;38(6):600–9.

11. Neal B, MacMahon S, Chapman N. Effects of ACE inhibitors, calcium antagonists, and other blood-pressure-lowering drugs: results of prospectively designed overviews of randomised trials. Blood Pressure Lowering Treatment Trialists' collaboration. Lancet 2000;356:1955–64.

12. Viera AJ, Hawes E. Management of mild hypertension in adults. BMJ 2016;355: i5719.

13. Jones DW, Appel LJ, Sheps SG, et al. Measuring blood pressure accurately: new and persistent challenges. JAMA 2003;289(8):1027–30.

14. Pickering TG, Hall JE, Appel LJ, et al. Recommendations for blood pressure measurement in humans and experimental animals: part 1: blood pressure measurement in humans: a statement for professionals from the subcommittee of professional and public education of the American Heart Association Council on High Blood Pressure Research. Circulation 2005;111(5):697–716.

15. Reeves RA. Does this patient have hypertension: how to measure blood pressure. JAMA 1995;273:1211–8.

16. Turner JR, Viera AJ, Shimbo D. Ambulatory blood pressure monitoring in clinical practice: a review. Am J Med 2015;128(1):14–20.

17. Myers MG, Valdivieso MA. Use of an automated blood pressure recording device, the BpTRU, to reduce the "white coat effect" in routine practice. Am J Hypertens 2003;16(6):494–7.

18. Leung AA, Nerenberg K, Daskalopoulou SS, et al. Hypertension Canada's 2016 Canadian hypertension education program guidelines for blood pressure measurement, diagnosis, assessment of risk, prevention, and treatment of hypertension. Can J Cardiol 2016;32(5):569–88.

19. Pickering TG, White WB, Giles TD, et al. When and how to use self (home) and ambulatory blood pressure monitoring. J Am Soc Hypertens 2010;4(2):56–61.

20. Verberk WJ, Kroon AA, Kessels AG, et al. Home blood pressure measurement: a systematic review. J Am Coll Cardiol 2005;46(5):743–51.

21. Stergiou GS, Salgami EV, Tzamouranis DG, et al. Masked hypertension assessed by ambulatory versus home blood pressure monitoring: is it the same phenomenon? Am J Hypertens 2005;18:772–8.

22. Verberk WJ, Kroon AA, Kessels AG, et al. The optimal scheme of self blood pressure measurement as determined from ambulatory blood pressure recordings. J Hypertens 2006;24(8):1541–8.

23. U.S. Preventive Services Task Force. Final Recommendation Statement. Hypertension in adults: screening and home monitoring. Available at: http://www.uspreventiveservicestaskforce.org/Page/Document/RecommendationStatementFinal/high-blood-pressure-in-adults-screening. Accessed November 28, 2016.

24. U.S. Preventive Services Task Force. Screening for high blood pressure: U.S. preventive services task force reaffirmation recommendation statement. AHRQ Pub. No. 08-15105-EF-3. December 2007. Ann Intern Med 2007;147:783–6.

25. Piper MA, Evans CV, Burda BU, et al. Diagnostic and predictive accuracy of blood pressure screening methods with consideration of rescreening intervals:

a systematic review for the U.S. Preventive Services Task Force. Ann Intern Med 2015;162(3):192–204.

26. Luehr D, Woolley T, Burke R, et al. Hypertension diagnosis and treatment. Bloomington (MN): Institute for Clinical Systems Improvement (ICSI); 2012. p. 67. Available at: http://www.guideline.gov/content.aspx?id=39321.

27. Perloff D, Sokolow M, Cowan R. The prognostic value of ambulatory blood pressures. JAMA 1983;249:2792–8.

28. Verdecchia P, Porcellati C, Schillaci G, et al. Ambulatory blood pressure: an independent predictor of prognosis in essential hypertension. Hypertension 1994;24:793–801.

29. Bjorklund K, Lind L, Zethelius B, et al. Prognostic significance of 24-h ambulatory blood pressure characteristics for cardiovascular morbidity in a population of elderly men. J Hypertens 2004;22:1691–7.

30. Sega R, Facchetti R, Bombelli M, et al. Prognostic value of ambulatory and home blood pressures compared with office blood pressure in the general population: follow-up results from the Pressione Arteriose Monitorate E Loro Associazioni (PAMELA) study. Circulation 2005;111:1777–83.

31. Staessen JA, Thijs L, Fagard R, et al. Predicting cardiovascular risk using conventional vs ambulatory blood pressure in older patients with systolic hypertension. JAMA 1999;282:539–46.

32. Dolan E, Stanton A, Thijs L, et al. Superiority of ambulatory over clinic blood pressure measurement in predicting mortality: the Dublin outcome study. Hypertension 2005;46:156–61.

33. Hodgkinson J, Mant J, Martin U, et al. Relative effectiveness of clinic and home blood pressure monitoring compared with ambulatory blood pressure monitoring in diagnosis of hypertension: systematic review. BMJ 2011;342:d3621.

34. Lovibond K, Jowett S, Barton P, et al. Cost-effectiveness of options for the diagnosis of high blood pressure in primary care: a modelling study. Lancet 2011; 378(9798):1219–30.

35. Franklin SS, Thijs L, Asayama K, et al, IDACO Investigators. The cardiovascular risk of white-coat hypertension. J Am Coll Cardiol 2016;68(19):2033–43.

36. James PA, Oparil S, Carter BL, et al. 2014 evidence-based guideline for the management of high blood pressure in adults: report from the panel members appointed to the Eighth Joint National Committee (JNC 8). JAMA 2014;311(5):507–20.

37. SPRINT Research Group, Wright JT Jr, Williamson JD, Whelton PK, et al. A randomized trial of intensive versus standard blood-pressure control. N Engl J Med 2015;373(22):2103–16.

38. Bress AP, Tanner RM, Hess R, et al. Generalizability of results from the Systolic Blood Pressure Intervention Trial (SPRINT) to the US adult population. J Am Coll Cardiol 2015. http://dx.doi.org/10.1016/j.jacc.2015.10.037.

39. Carol JJ, Salas M, Speckman JL, et al. Persistence with treatment for hypertension in actual practice. CMAJ 1999;160:31–7.

40. O'Connor PJ, Sperl-Hillen JM, Johnson PE, et al. Clinical inertia and outpatient medical errors. Available at: http://www.ahrq.gov/downloads/pub/advances/vol2/oconnor.pdf. Accessed November 28, 2016.

41. Walsh JM, McDonald KM, Shojania KG, et al. Quality improvement strategies for hypertension management: a systematic review. Med Care 2006;44(7):646–57.

42. Jaffe MG, Lee GA, Young JD, et al. Improved blood pressure control associated with a large-scale hypertension program. JAMA 2013;310(7):699–705.

43. Walsh JM, Sundaram V, McDonald K, et al. Implementing effective hypertension quality improvement strategies: barriers and potential solutions. J Clin Hypertens (Greenwich) 2008;10:311–6.

Aspirin for Primary Prevention

Ilana B. Richman, MD[a],*, Douglas K. Owens, MD, MS[b,c]

KEYWORDS

- Aspirin • Cardiovascular disease prevention • Colorectal cancer prevention
- Guidelines

KEY POINTS

- Studies of aspirin for primary prevention of cardiovascular disease suggest an approximate 22% reduction in risk of nonfatal myocardial infarction and for stroke, by approximately 14%.
- Aspirin use likely reduces risk of colorectal cancer and colorectal cancer mortality, although time to benefit is long (10–20 years).
- Aspirin increases the risk of gastrointestinal bleeding and hemorrhagic stroke, although both are uncommon events. There are no prospectively validated tools to assess bleeding risk.
- A recent mathematical modeling study incorporated cardiovascular disease and colorectal cancer benefits with bleeding risks; the greatest net benefit was seen among adults 50 to 59 with moderate to high cardiovascular risk.
- Updated US Preventive Services Task Force guidelines recommend aspirin for the primary prevention of cardiovascular disease and colorectal cancer among adults 50 to 59 who are at increased cardiovascular risk.

INTRODUCTION

Salicylates have been used since antiquity to alleviate pain, fever, and inflammation. It was not until the mid 20th century, though, that physicians recognized aspirin's antithrombotic properties and began to use aspirin to prevent myocardial infarction (MI).[1] In

Disclosures: Dr I.B. Richman was supported by a VA Health Services Research and Development fellowship during the initial drafting of this review. Dr D.K. Owens was supported by the Department of Veterans Affairs. He was a member of the US Preventive Services Task Force. The views expressed in this article are those of the authors and do not necessarily reflect the position nor the policy of the Department of Veterans Affairs or the US Preventive Services Task Force.

a Department of Medicine, Yale University School of Medicine, 367 Cedar Street, Harkness Hall A, Room 301, New Haven, CT 06510, USA; b VA Palo Alto Health Care System, Palo Alto, CA, USA; c Department of Medicine, Stanford University School of Medicine, Center for Primary Care and Outcomes Research/Center for Health Policy, 117 Encina Commons, Stanford, CA 94305, USA
* Corresponding author.
E-mail address: ilana.richman@yale.edu

Med Clin N Am 101 (2017) 713–724
http://dx.doi.org/10.1016/j.mcna.2017.03.004

the 1970s, insights into the cell biology of cancer led to the hypothesis that aspirin might also be an effective chemotherapeutic or chemopreventive agent.[2,3] Following these observations, a number of landmark clinical trials have evaluated aspirin for both the prevention of cardiovascular disease and cancer.

Today, aspirin continues to be widely used, particularly for cardiovascular disease prevention. Among adults 45 to 75 in the United States, 52% report taking aspirin daily. Daily aspirin use is common even among those who do not have a history of heart disease (47%).[4] Despite its popularity, aspirin for cardiovascular disease prevention has been controversial. In 2014, The Food and Drug Administration (FDA) advised that current evidence does not support the routine use of aspirin for primary prevention of heart attack or stroke.[5] The statement cited weak evidence for benefit for cardiovascular disease prevention as well as potential for harm from bleeding.

In contrast, the US Preventive Services Task Force (USPSTF) recently issued guidelines endorsing aspirin's use for primary prevention of cardiovascular disease and colorectal cancer in specific populations.[6] The USPSTF is an independent committee composed of experts who regularly review the medical literature and compile evidence-based recommendations for preventive service use in primary care. In 2016, the USPSTF recommended low-dose aspirin for the prevention of colorectal cancer and cardiovascular disease among adults ages 50 to 59 who have 10-year risk of at least 10% for cardiovascular disease. The USPSTF stated that adults 60 to 69 who have 10-year risk of at least a 10% for cardiovascular disease may also benefit, but the decision to initiate aspirin in that age group should be individualized. The task force's recommendations are summarized in **Table 1**.

To estimate 10-year cardiovascular risk, the USPSTF recommended using the American College of Cardiology/American Heart Association Atherosclerotic Cardiovascular Disease (ASCVD) risk calculator.[7] The patient characteristics used to estimate cardiovascular risk are described in **Box 1** and calculators are freely accessible online (http://tools.acc.org/ASCVD-Risk-Estimator/).[8] The risk calculator has several advantages including that it has been validated in US populations;

Table 1
Summary of USPSTF recommendations

Population	Recommendation	Grade
Adults ages 50–59, ≥10% 10-y CVD risk	Initiate low-dose aspirin use.	B (The USPSTF recommends the service. There is moderate certainty that the benefit is moderate to substantial.)
Adults ages 60–69, ≥10% 10-y CVD risk	The decision to initiate low-dose aspirin use is an individual one.	C (At least moderate certainty that there is a small net benefit. USPSTF recommends selectively offering aspirin to individual patients based on professional judgment and patient preferences.)
Adults ages 40–49	No recommendation.	I (The USPTF concludes that the current evidence is insufficient to assess the balance of benefits and harms of the service).
Adults ages ≥ 70	No recommendation.	I (The USPTF concludes that the current evidence is insufficient to assess the balance of benefits and harms of the service.)

Abbreviations: CVD, cardiovascular disease; USPSTF, US Preventive Services Task Force.

| **Box 1** |
| **Atherosclerotic cardiovascular disease risk calculator variables** |
| • Gender |
| • Age |
| • High-density lipoprotein cholesterol |
| • Total cholesterol |
| • Diabetes mellitus |
| • Treatment for hypertension |
| • Race |
| • Systolic blood pressure |
| • Current smoker |

provides age-, sex-, and race-specific estimates of cardiovascular risk; and includes ischemic stroke as an outcome. However, several studies suggest the calculator may overestimate the risk of cardiovascular disease in modern, diverse patient popula-tions.[9,10] Although it is the best available tool currently for estimating risk in US pop-ulations, clinicians should be aware of the limitations and imprecision of all such tools.

The task force also advised that aspirin should be avoided in adults who are at high risk of bleeding, who have a limited life expectancy, or who do not want to take a daily aspirin. The recommendation statement noted that there is insufficient evidence to recommend for or against initiating aspirin among adults 40 to 49 or adults 70 and older and that continuing aspirin in adults over age 70 is an individualized decision.[6]

What informed the USPSTF's recommendations and why did they differ from the FDA's assessment of aspirin? One major difference between the 2 approaches is that the USPSTF considered aspirin's role in preventing cardiovascular disease and cancer together, whereas the FDA considered only cardiovascular disease benefits. To evaluate aspirin's benefits in 2 distinct disease areas (cancer and cardiovascular disease) as well as its harms, the USPSTF took a 2-step approach. First, the USPSTF commissioned 3 separate metaanalyses of available data on aspirin for the primary prevention of cardiovascular disease, prevention of cancer including colorectal can-cer, and risk of major bleeding. Second, the task force commissioned a study that used data from these metaanalyses and other sources in a decision model designed to evaluate the net balance of benefits and harms of aspirin in different populations. In this review, we summarize the findings that informed the USPSTF's recommendations and explore key areas of uncertainty in aspirin for primary prevention.

ASPIRIN AND PRIMARY PREVENTION OF CARDIOVASCULAR DISEASE
Nonfatal Myocardial Infarction

Nearly 30 years ago, the British Doctors Trial first evaluated whether aspirin can pre-vent MI. The trial, which randomized healthy male physicians to aspirin, reported a nonsignificant 3% reduction in the rate of nonfatal MI.[11] One year later, though, the Physicians' Health Study, an analogous but larger trial conducted in the United States, reported a significant reduction in nonfatal MI (hazard ratio, 0.59; 95% confidence in-terval [CI], 0.47–0.74).[12]

Since those early studies, a total of 10 high-quality trials have evaluated aspirin for the primary prevention of MI.[13] Echoing the pattern of those initial studies, the

USPSTF's metaanalysis found substantial heterogeneity among these trials (I^2 62%). Overall, however, the metaanalysis reported a reduction in the relative risk (RR) of nonfatal MI among those taking aspirin (RR, 0.78; 95% CI, 0.71–0.87). Three of the 4 largest trials included in the metaanalysis demonstrated benefit, and the fourth demonstrated benefit among older participants. Taken together, these results suggest that aspirin does reduce the risk of nonfatal MI.

Although these findings support aspirin's efficacy, aspirin's absolute benefit in reducing nonfatal MI is modest. Given the typical rates of MI seen among patients enrolled in primary prevention trials, low-dose aspirin would prevent about 4 to 5 nonfatal heart attacks for every 1000 people treated with aspirin for 10 years.[13] Aspirin's cardiovascular disease benefits appear early on after initiating use, likely within the first 1 to 5 years of use.[13]

Nonfatal Stroke

Aspirin's antiplatelet properties suggest that aspirin may both lower the risk of ischemic stroke and increase the risk of hemorrhagic stroke. The USPSTF's metaanalysis examined 10 trials that reported both ischemic and hemorrhagic stroke outcomes. Across aspirin trials, hemorrhagic stroke accounted for only about 16% of strokes.[14] Combining these 10 trials, there was no evidence that aspirin reduced stroke risk (RR, 0.95; 95% CI, 0.85–1.06).[13] Among the 7 trials that used only low-dose aspirin (<100 mg/d), however, the metaanalysis found a reduction in the risk of nonfatal stroke (RR, 0.86; 95% CI, 0.76–0.98.). In primary prevention trials, aspirin did seem to increase the risk of hemorrhagic stroke (odds ratio [OR], 1.33; 95% CI, 1.03–1.71).[14] Even low-dose aspirin may increase the risk of hemorrhagic stroke, although the estimate from the USPSTF metaanalysis did not attain statistical significance (OR, 1.27; 95% CI, 0.96–1.68).[14]

As with prevention of MI, the absolute risk reduction in stroke is modest. Given the typical stroke rates seen in primary prevention trials, low-dose aspirin would prevent about 4 nonfatal strokes for every 1000 people treated for 10 years.[13]

Cardiovascular Death

Across 11 trials, a pooled analysis did not demonstrate a statistically significant reduction in risk of cardiovascular death (RR, 0.94; 95% CI, 0.86–1.03).[13]

Special Populations and Effect Modification

Is aspirin especially beneficial in any particular population? Aspirin prevents more cardiovascular events among patients who are more likely to have cardiovascular events. Thus, the greater the underlying risk, the greater the absolute benefit. For example, among patients enrolled in primary prevention trials, there was a near 10-fold difference in the estimated absolute benefit, depending on baseline risk. For those with the lowest cardiovascular disease risk, aspirin prevented approximately 0.15 nonfatal MIs per 1000 person-years compared with and 1.43 MIs per 1000 person-years in the highest risk populations.[13]

The benefits of aspirin may vary with age, and in particular, the RR reduction for MI may increase with age.[13] Three trials that reported results by age demonstrated larger RR reductions for MI at older ages, although not all trials reported significant interactions.[12,15,16] Several trials also evaluated stroke rates with aspirin use by age and did not show significant differences, although event rates were low in subgroup analyses.[13]

A previous metaanalysis examined effects of aspirin on stroke and MI risk by sex and reported larger reductions in MI for men and greater reductions in stroke risk for women with aspirin use, although the study did not assess for sex-specific interactions specifically.[17] These sex-specific differences were largely driven by findings from the Women's Health Study, which reported a reduction in stroke but not MI with aspirin use in women.[15] Overall, though, owing to inconsistency across trials, lack of subgroup prespecification, and lack of formal interaction testing, the USPSTF concluded there was not sufficient evidence to support differences in the effect of aspirin by sex for the combined outcome of cardiovascular disease.

A number of trials have evaluated aspirin's specific cardiovascular effects in patients with diabetes.[12,15,18] Results from these trials did not suggest effect modification for risk of stroke or MI among patients with diabetes.

ASPIRIN AND CANCER

In addition to its antiplatelet effects, aspirin has recognized antineoplastic properties. A number of dedicated trials have demonstrated aspirin's effectiveness in reducing colonic adenomas, although these trials focused on precancerous lesions.[19,20] Reanalysis of cardiovascular disease prevention trials has provided some insight into aspirin's effect on the development of colorectal cancer and death from colorectal cancer.

Data from cardiovascular disease prevention trials suggest that regular aspirin use reduces the incidence of colorectal cancer by about 40% (RR, 0.60; 95% CI, 0.47–0.76).[21] This benefit is seen between 10 and 20 years after initiating aspirin. Within 10 years of initiation, aspirin has little benefit (RR, 0.99; 95% CI, 0.85–1.15).[21] The minimum duration of aspirin use needed to reduce the risk of cancer is not well-established, but some data suggest that longer use is associated with greater benefit.[22] Given typical rates of cancer in the United States, and given the time required to see benefit, for every 1000 adults treated from age 50 onward, an estimated 12 to 14 cases of colorectal cancer could be prevented.[6,23] When used consistently for several years, aspirin also seems to reduce the risk of death from colorectal cancer (hazard ratio, 0.51; 95% CI, 0.35–0.74), although benefits only accrue after 10 to 20 years of initiation.[24]

In addition to colorectal cancer, the USPSTF evaluated aspirin's effect on incidence of all cancers. The metaanalysis examined 6 trials of aspirin for cardiovascular disease prevention and did not find a benefit (RR, 0.98; 95% CI, 0.93–1.04). When restricted to trials with a median intended duration of use of at least 4 years, there was a marginally statistically significant reduction in incidence of all cancers (RR, 0.86; 95% CI, 0.74–0.99). A metaanalysis of individual patient data from studies of aspirin for primary prevention reported a reduction in incidence of all cancers (hazard ratio, 0.88;, 95% CI, 0.80–0.98), with benefits seen 3 to 4 years after randomization.[25] This metaanalysis, however, included studies that only reported fatal cancers and also included studies of aspirin and warfarin coadministration.

The USPSTF metaanalysis also examined whether aspirin use reduces mortality from all cancers. In considering 10 trials that evaluated aspirin for primary prevention of cardiovascular disease, the metaanalysis did not demonstrate a reduction in cancer deaths (RR, 0.96; 95% CI, 0.87–1.06). A previous metaanalysis had demonstrated a reduction in cancer death after at least 4 years of use (hazard ratio, 0.82; 95% CI, 0.70–0.95), although that analysis excluded trials of alternate day dosing and included trials of high-dose aspirin unlikely to be used for primary prevention of cardiovascular disease.[24]

ASPIRIN AND BLEEDING COMPLICATIONS

Although aspirin's antithrombotic properties reduce heart attack and ischemic stroke, those same properties can promote bleeding, including disabling or life-threatening central nervous system bleeding. In addition, aspirin promotes gastric ulcer formation, which, in turn, creates additional risk for bleeding.

The USPSTF commissioned a metaanalysis specifically to synthesize evidence on bleeding risks, particularly gastrointestinal (GI) bleeding and hemorrhagic stroke, the most serious forms of bleeding. The metaanalysis found that, overall, GI bleeding is rare, with less than 1% of those on aspirin affected. Still, aspirin is associated with GI bleeding (OR, 1.59; 95% CI, 1.32–1.91) and even low-dose aspirin seems to increase risk (OR, 1.58; 95% CI 1.29–1.95).[14] Although these point estimates were similar, observational studies suggest that higher doses are associated with a higher risk of GI bleeding.[26] Depending on the underlying risk of bleeding, aspirin might be expected to contribute between 1 and 6 cases of GI bleeding for every 1000 adults treated for 10 years.[14]

A number of individual risk factors affect bleeding risk (**Box 2**). Trials of aspirin for cardiovascular disease prevention have identified a number of risk factors including age, male sex, diabetes, hypertension, tobacco use, and obesity as risk factors for bleeding.[14] A number of other conditions, including advanced liver and renal disease and concurrent use of other anticoagulants, can also increase the risk of bleeding. Trials have generally not compared doses of aspirin, but observational data suggest that risk of both GI and central nervous system bleeding increases with dose.[26,27] Although there are known risk factors for bleeding that may help to qualitatively risk stratify patients, there have been no prospectively validated tools for predicting bleeding risk among those taking aspirin.

MODELING TO UNDERSTAND THE BENEFITS AND HARMS OF ASPIRIN

Should we recommend aspirin for primary prevention to our patients? Aspirin reduces nonfatal MI, ischemic stroke, and mortality from colorectal cancer but increases GI and intracranial bleeding. Weighing these benefits and harms, however, may not be straightforward, especially when the risks and benefits may vary according to population and time frame. One way to quantitatively evaluate the net benefit of aspirin is to use decision modeling.[28–30]

Box 2
Risk factors for bleeding when considering aspirin initiation

- Demographics
  - Older age
  - Male sex

- Medical history
  - Diabetes mellitus
  - Hypertension
  - Liver disease
  - Renal disease
  - Previous hospitalization for gastrointestinal problem or history of abdominal pain
  - Thrombocytopenia or underlying coagulopathy
  - Obesity

- Aspirin properties and medication interactions
  - Dose and duration of use
  - Use of nonsteroidal antiinflammatory drugs
  - Anticoagulant use
  - Tobacco use

Decision models are a methodologic approach for estimating the effects of interventions on health outcomes in different populations over time.[29] Modeling is especially useful for a treatment like aspirin, in which risks and benefits vary by patient and where risks and benefits appear at different time points. A related advantage of modeling is that it allows us to quantify aspirin's overall impact on quantity and quality of life. Even if we knew the number of patients who might be expected to benefit or be harmed by aspirin, comparing those outcomes is difficult if each has a different severity and impact on quality of life. Modeling addresses this by translating outcomes into a single measure, the quality-adjusted life-year, which incorporates both duration and quality of life.[31] Because the main effect of aspirin is on nonfatal events, which can substantially decrease quality of life, the use of QALYs is particularly helpful for assessing the usefulness of aspirin.

Using this approach, investigators working with the USPSTF developed a decision model of aspirin for the primary prevention of colorectal cancer and cardiovascular disease.[23] The main modeling results are reported in **Table 2**. The analysis found that benefits generally outweighed harms and were greatest for men and women who initiate aspirin in their 50s and continue until death or an adverse event. Benefits increased as risk of cardiovascular disease increased. For example, men in their 50s with a 10-year risk of 10% of cardiovascular disease would gain a net 58.8 QALYs per 1000 adults treated over a lifetime, whereas men with a 20% risk of cardiovascular disease would gain 83.4 QALYs.[6,23]

One final advantage of modeling is its ability to ask "what if" questions that build on the literature, but are not directly addressed in any clinical trial. For example, the modeling study addressed whether starting aspirin at a younger age, between 40 and 49 years, is beneficial. The model results suggested initiating aspirin in this age range provides the greatest benefit, although these results rely on extrapolating aspirin's benefits to this younger population, because this younger population has not been the focus of clinical trials. The USPSTF did not recommend aspirin use in younger patients because of the lack of empirical evidence.

The results from the modeling study should be interpreted with an understanding of the strengths and limitations of modeling. First, models rely on the best available estimates of effect from the literature. A strength of this analysis is that the model incorporated results from the 3 comprehensive metaanalyses discussed herein and from additional evidence. However, if there are unidentified biases in these estimates from the literature, they will be reflected in the model results. Second, models require making choices about which benefits and harms to include, and those choices can affect the model's estimates. For example, in the accompanying metaanalysis, risk of hemorrhagic stroke with low-dose aspirin was not statistically significant (OR, 1.27; 95% CI, 0.96–1.68), but was still incorporated in the main model, largely because the authors felt that the point estimate represented a real effect.[23] A sensitivity analysis excluding this risk favored aspirin more strongly. Readers should appreciate that all models require simplifying a complex reality through a set of choices and these choices can influence the model's findings. The substantial advantage of modeling is that it provides an approach for estimating net benefit when there are complex benefits and harms.

AREAS OF UNCERTAINTY AND FUTURE CONSIDERATIONS
Dose

Of the 11 cardiovascular disease primary prevention trials, 8 included in the USPSTF metaanalysis used a dose of 100 mg of aspirin or less. A dose of 81 mg is commonly

Table 2
Lifetime benefits, harms, and net benefit of aspirin per 10,000 men and women by age group and baseline 10-y CVD risk

CVD Risk[a]	Nonfatal MIs Prevented	Nonfatal Ischemic Strokes Prevented	Colorectal Cancer Cases Prevented	Serious GI Bleeding Events Caused	Hemorrhagic Strokes Caused	Net Life-Years Gained	QALYs Gained
Men							
50–59 y							
10%	225	84	139	284	23	333	588
15%	267	86	121	260	28	395	644
20%	286	92	122	248	21	605	834
60–69 y							
10%	159	66	112	314	31	–20	180
15%	186	80	104	298	24	96	309
20%	201	84	91	267	27	116	318
Women							
50–59 y							
10%	148	137	139	209	35	219	621
15%	150	143	135	200	34	334	716
20%	152	144	132	184	29	463	833
60–69 y							
10%	101	116	105	230	32	–12	284
15%	110	129	93	216	34	17	324
20%	111	130	97	217	33	48	360

Abbreviations: CVD, cardiovascular disease; GI, gastrointestinal; MI, myocardial infarction; QALY, quality-adjusted life-year; USPSTF, US Preventive Services Task Force

[a] The 10-y CVD risk is based on the American College of Cardiology/American Heart Association risk calculator estimate.

Adapted from Bibbins-Domingo K. Aspirin use for the primary prevention of cardiovascular disease and colorectal cancer: US Preventive Services Task Force recommendation statement. Ann Intern Med 2016;164(12):839; with permission.

prescribed in the United States. There are no trials, though, that specifically compare doses head-to-head for primary prevention, although studies are underway.[13]

Is low-dose aspirin preferable? Bleeding may be lower with lower doses. Although there are very few direct comparisons of dose for primary prevention, observational data suggest a higher risk of both GI and intracranial bleeding with increased doses.[26,27] Second, the reduction in ischemic stroke is based on trials with dosages of less than 100 mg.[13] In contrast, some evidence suggests higher doses have a more potent antineoplastic effect.[24] The available evidence seems to suggest that a dose of less than100 mg/d provides the best balance of risk and benefit for primary prevention.[6]

Age

Most trials of aspirin for primary prevention of cardiovascular disease included participants in their 50s and 60s. Although some trials did include older and younger patients, these trials either did not report age-specific findings, were not powered to detect age-specific effects, or did not look at the extremes of age.[12,32,33] Although the USPSTF modeling study suggested that taking aspirin beginning at that younger age may produce the greatest benefit, the direct evidence underlying this result is sparse. Similarly, there is no randomized trial evidence to guide aspirin initiation among adults over the age of 70, although aspirin use is quite common in this population. Although cardiovascular disease risk increases with advancing age, bleeding risk also increases, and the balance of risks and benefits is less clear. There is ongoing research to evaluate the benefit of initiating aspirin in adults over the age of 70.[34]

Other Cancers

Previous metaanalyses have suggested that aspirin may indeed reduce incidence and death from cancers other than colorectal cancer.[24,25] These metaanalyses, however, included studies that are difficult to generalize to a primary prevention population. For example, the metaanalyses included studies that used higher doses of aspirin, excluded studies of every-other-day dosing or coadministered aspirin and warfarin. Despite this uncertainty, these metaanalyses offer some evidence that aspirin may have a role in reducing risk from cancers other than colorectal cancer.

SUMMARY

Current evidence supports initiating aspirin for primary prevention in selected higher risk populations. In particular, adults in their 50s who are at increased risk of cardiovascular disease and are not at increased risk of bleeding are most likely to benefit. Adults in their 60s may also benefit, although the risk of harm increases with age. Older populations are also less likely to benefit from colorectal cancer risk reduction, as this benefit takes years to manifest. In general, treatment decisions should involve an assessment of the individual's risk of cardiovascular disease, bleeding risk, and life expectancy. Incorporating patient preferences is also critical in deciding whether to initiate aspirin for primary prevention.

When evaluating an intervention with complex benefits and harms such as aspirin, decision modeling provides a useful approach. The modeling integrated evidence about the effect of aspirin on cardiovascular and colorectal cancer outcomes. Based on the evidence reviews and modeling, the USPSTF concluded that aspirin's benefits outweigh its harms in specific populations. These conclusions differ from the FDA's recommendations, in part because the USPSTF considered the benefits of aspirin for both cardiovascular disease and cancer, whereas the FDA focused on cardiovascular benefits alone.

Decades of research on aspirin have refined our understanding of its benefits and risks. Current evidence supports the use of aspirin for primary prevention in specific populations. Ongoing studies will likely help further define the optimal dose of aspirin, its use in broader age groups, and its role in prevention of other cancers.

REFERENCES

1. Miner J, Hoffhines A. The discovery of aspirin's antithrombotic effects. Tex Heart Inst J 2007;34(2):179–86. Available at: http://www.ncbi.nlm.nih.gov/pubmed/17622365. Accessed October 11, 2016.
2. Gasic G, Gasic T, Murphy S. Anti-metastatic effect of aspirin. Lancet 1972; 300(7783):932–3.
3. Vainio H, Morgan G, Kleihues P. An international evaluation of the cancer-preventive potential of nonsteroidal anti-inflammatory drugs. Cancer Epidemiol Biomarkers Prev 1997;6(9):749–53. Available at: http://www.ncbi.nlm.nih.gov/pubmed/9298584. Accessed September 1, 2016.
4. Williams CD, Chan AT, Elman MR, et al. Aspirin use among adults in the U.S.: results of a national survey. Am J Prev Med 2015;48(5):501–8. Available at: http://www.ncbi.nlm.nih.gov/pubmed/25891049. Accessed October 11, 2016.
5. US Food and Drug Administration. Information for consumers (drugs): use of aspirin for primary prevention of heart attack and stroke. Available at: https://www.fda.gov/Drugs/ResourcesForYou/Consumers/ucm390574.htm. Accessed March 17, 2017.
6. Aspirin use for the primary prevention of cardiovascular disease and colorectal cancer: recommendations from the U.S. Preventive Services Task Force. Ann Intern Med 2016;164(12):836–45. Available at: http://annals.org/article.aspx?doi=10.7326/P16-9015. Accessed October 11, 2016.
7. Goff DC Jr, Lloyd-Jones DM, Bennett G, et al. 2013 ACC/AHA guideline on the assessment of cardiovascular risk. Circulation 2014;129(25 Suppl 2):S49–73.
8. ASCVD risk estimator. Available at: http://tools.acc.org/ASCVD-Risk-Estimator/. Accessed October 11, 2016.
9. Rana JS, Tabada GH, Solomon MD, et al. Accuracy of the atherosclerotic cardiovascular risk equation in a large contemporary, multiethnic population. J Am Coll Cardiol 2016;67(18):2118–30. Available at: http://linkinghub.elsevier.com/retrieve/pii/S0735109716010251. Accessed November 18, 2016.
10. DeFilippis AP, Young R, Carrubba CJ, et al. An analysis of calibration and discrimination among multiple cardiovascular risk scores in a modern multiethnic cohort. Ann Intern Med 2015;162(4):266. Available at: http://annals.org/article.aspx?doi=10.7326/M14-1281. Accessed November 18, 2016.
11. Peto R, Gray R, Collins R, et al. Randomised trial of prophylactic daily aspirin in British male doctors. Br Med J (Clin Res Ed) 1988;296(6618):313–6. Available at: http://www.ncbi.nlm.nih.gov/pubmed/3125882. Accessed June 23, 2016.
12. Final report on the aspirin component of the ongoing physicians' health study. Steering committee of the physicians' health study research group. N Engl J Med 1989;321(3):129–35. Available at: http://www.nejm.org/doi/abs/10.1056/NEJM198907203210301. Accessed January 15, 2017.
13. Guirguis-Blake JM, Evans CV, Senger CA, et al. Aspirin for the primary prevention of cardiovascular events: a systematic evidence review for the U.S. Preventive

Services Task Force. Ann Intern Med 2016;164(12):804–13. Available at: http://www.ncbi.nlm.nih.gov/pubmed/27064410. Accessed June 23, 2016.

14. Whitlock EP, Burda BU, Williams SB, et al. Bleeding risks with aspirin use for primary prevention in adults: a systematic review for the U.S. Preventive Services Task Force. Ann Intern Med 2016;164(12):826–35. Available at: http://www.ncbi.nlm.nih.gov/pubmed/27064261. Accessed June 24, 2016.

15. Ridker PM, Cook NR, Lee IM, et al. A randomized trial of low-dose aspirin in the primary prevention of cardiovascular disease in women. N Engl J Med 2005;352(13):1293–304. Available at: http://www.nejm.org/doi/abs/10.1056/NEJMoa050613. Accessed October 20, 2016.

16. Kjeldsen SE, Kolloch RE, Leonetti G, et al. Influence of gender and age on preventing cardiovascular disease by antihypertensive treatment and acetylsalicylic acid. The HOT study. Hypertension optimal treatment. J Hypertens 2000; 18(5):629–42. Available at: http://www.ncbi.nlm.nih.gov/pubmed/10826567. Accessed January 15, 2017.

17. Berger JS, Roncaglioni MC, Avanzini F, et al. Aspirin for the primary prevention of cardiovascular events in women and men. JAMA 2006; 295(3):306. Available at: http://www.ncbi.nlm.nih.gov/pubmed/16418466. Accessed January 15, 2017.

18. Sacco M, Pellegrini F, Roncaglioni MC, et al. Primary prevention of cardiovascular events with low-dose aspirin and vitamin E in type 2 diabetic patients. Diabetes Care 2003;26(12):3264–72.

19. Baron JA, Cole BF, Sandler RS, et al. A randomized trial of aspirin to prevent colorectal adenomas. N Engl J Med 2003;348(10):891–9. Available at: http://www.nejm.org/doi/abs/10.1056/NEJMoa021735. Accessed October 17, 2016.

20. Sandler RS, Halabi S, Baron JA, et al. A randomized trial of aspirin to prevent colorectal adenomas in patients with previous colorectal cancer. N Engl J Med 2003;348(10):883–90. Available at: http://www.nejm.org/doi/abs/10.1056/NEJMoa021633. Accessed October 17, 2016.

21. Chubak J, Whitlock EP, Williams SB, et al. Aspirin for the prevention of cancer incidence and mortality: systematic evidence reviews for the U.S. Preventive Services Task Force. Ann Intern Med 2016;164(12):814–25. Available at: http://www.ncbi.nlm.nih.gov/pubmed/27064482. Accessed June 23, 2016.

22. Chubak J, Kamineni A , Buist DSM, et al. Aspirin Use for the Prevention of Colorectal Cancer: An Updated Systematic Evidence Review for the U.S. Preventive Services Task Force. Evidence Synthesis No. 133. AHRQ Publication No. 15-05228-EF-1. Rockville (MD). Agency for Healthcare Research and Quality. Available at: https://www.ncbi.nlm.nih.gov/pubmed/26491758. Accessed September, 2015.

23. Dehmer SP, Maciosek MV, Flottemesch TJ, et al. Aspirin for the primary prevention of cardiovascular disease and colorectal cancer: a decision analysis for the U.S. Preventive Services Task Force. Ann Intern Med 2016;164(12): 777–86. Available at: http://annals.org/article.aspx?doi=10.7326/M15-2129. Accessed November 22, 2016.

24. Rothwell PM, Fowkes FG, Belch JF, et al. Effect of daily aspirin on long-term risk of death due to cancer: analysis of individual patient data from randomised trials. Lancet 2011;377(9759):31–41. Available at: http://www.ncbi.nlm.nih.gov/pubmed/21144578. Accessed August 2, 2016.

25. Rothwell PM, Price JF, Fowkes FG, et al. Short-term effects of daily aspirin on cancer incidence, mortality, and non-vascular death: analysis of the time course of risks and benefits in 51 randomised controlled trials. Lancet 2012;379(9826):

1602–12. Available at: http://www.ncbi.nlm.nih.gov/pubmed/22440946. Accessed October 20, 2016.

26. Huang ES, Strate LL, Ho WW, et al. Long-term use of aspirin and the risk of gastrointestinal bleeding. Am J Med 2011;124(5):426–33. Available at: http://linkinghub.elsevier.com/retrieve/pii/S0002934311000957. Accessed October 11, 2016.

27. Iso H, Hennekens CH, Stampfer MJ, et al. Prospective study of aspirin use and risk of stroke in women. Stroke 1999;30(9):1764–71. Available at: http://www.ncbi.nlm.nih.gov/pubmed/10471421. Accessed October 11, 2016.

28. Habbema JD, Wilt TJ, Etzioni R, et al. Models in the development of clinical practice guidelines. Ann Intern Med 2014;161(11):812. Available at: http://annals.org/article.aspx?doi=10.7326/M14-0845. Accessed November 18, 2016.

29. Owens DK, Whitlock EP, Henderson J, et al. Use of decision models in the development of evidence-based clinical preventive services recommendations: methods of the U.S. Preventive Services Task Force. Ann Intern Med 2016; 165(7):501–8. Available at: http://annals.org/article.aspx?doi=10.7326/M15-2531. Accessed November 18, 2016.

30. Neumann PJ, Russell LB, Sanders GD, et al. Cost-effectiveness in health and medicine. Available at: https://global.oup.com/academic/product/cost-effectiveness-in-health-and-medicine-9780190492939?cc=us&lang=en&.

31. Weinstein MC, Torrance G, McGuire A. QALYs: the basics. Value Health 2009; 12(Suppl 1):S5–9. Available at: http://linkinghub.elsevier.com/retrieve/pii/S1098301510600460. Accessed October 20, 2016.

32. Ogawa H, Nakayama M, Morimoto T, et al. Low-dose aspirin for primary prevention of atherosclerotic events in patients with type 2 diabetes: a randomized controlled trial. JAMA 2008;300(18):2134–41. Available at: http://www.ncbi.nlm.nih.gov/pubmed/18997198. Accessed January 25, 2017.

33. Hansson L, Zanchetti A, Carruthers SG, et al. Effects of intensive blood-pressure lowering and low-dose aspirin in patients with hypertension: principal results of the hypertension optimal treatment (HOT) randomised trial. HOT study group. Lancet 1998;351(9118):1755–62. Available at: http://www.ncbi.nlm.nih.gov/pubmed/9635947. Accessed October 20, 2016.

34. Aspirin in Reducing Events in the Elderly (ASPREE) | National Institute on Aging. Available at: https://www.nia.nih.gov/alzheimers/clinical-trials/aspirin-reducing-events-elderly-aspree. Accessed March 31, 2017.

Risk-based Breast Cancer Screening

Implications of Breast Density

Christoph I. Lee, MD, MS[a,b,c,*,1], Linda E. Chen, MD[a],
Joann G. Elmore, MD, MPH[d,e]

KEYWORDS

- Risk-based screening • Mammography • Breast density • Supplemental screening

KEY POINTS

- Breast density is just one factor that should be considered when physicians discuss risk-based breast cancer screening options with women.
- Digital mammography remains the primary screening tool for women with dense breasts.
- Based on early evidence, digital breast tomosynthesis, or three-dimensional mammography, may hold promise for improving screening accuracy among women with dense breasts, although studies are ongoing.
- Most women with dense breasts and no other risk factors are likely to experience more harms than benefits with supplemental screening ultrasonography.
- Women with dense breasts and additional risk factors that place them at high lifetime risk for developing breast cancer (>20%) should undergo breast MRI rather than supplemental screening ultrasonography.

Funding: C.I. Lee is supported by grants from the National Cancer Institute (grant P01CA154292) and American Cancer Society (grant 126947-MRSG-14-160-01-CPHPS). Dr J.G. Elmore is supported by a grant from the National Cancer Institute (R01 CA172343).
Disclosure: Dr C.I. Lee previously received research grants from GE Healthcare.
[a] Department of Radiology, University of Washington School of Medicine, 1959 Northeast Pacific Street, Seattle, WA 98195, USA; [b] Department of Health Services, University of Washington School of Public Health, 1959 Northeast Pacific Street, Seattle, WA 98195, USA; [c] Hutchinson Institute for Cancer Outcomes Research, Fred Hutchinson Research Cancer Center, 1100 Fairview Avenue N, Box 19024, Seattle, WA 98109, USA; [d] Department of Medicine, University of Washington School of Medicine, 325 Ninth Avenue, Box 359780, Seattle, WA 98104, USA; [e] Department of Epidemiology, University of Washington School of Public Health, 325 Ninth Avenue, Box 359780, Seattle, WA 98104, USA
[1] Present address: 617 Eastlake Avenue East, Seattle, WA 98109.
* Corresponding author. Seattle Cancer Care Alliance, 825 Eastlake Avenue East, G3-200, Seattle, WA 98109-1023.
E-mail address: stophlee@uw.edu

Med Clin N Am 101 (2017) 725–741
http://dx.doi.org/10.1016/j.mcna.2017.03.005

INTRODUCTION

With the recently revised recommendations for routine mammography screening from both the US Preventive Services Task Force (USPSTF) and the American Cancer Society (ACS),[1,2] there is growing consensus in the medical community that screening regimens should be tailored to patient risk. Overall, routine mammography screening has been shown to reduce mortality and, for patients at average risk, routine screening should begin around age 45 or 50 years. However, for those at increased risk, the start age and screening interval remain uncertain. Moreover, the increasing availability of new screening modalities beyond mammography further complicates the landscape of breast cancer screening.

Patient advocacy groups have brought personalized, risk-based screening to the forefront, focusing on breast density as a common risk factor for developing breast cancer. Given the widespread press coverage regarding breast density and a growing number of US state-level density reporting laws, women are increasingly bringing their questions about density as a risk factor to primary care physicians. Common concerns include the accuracy of screening mammography and whether they should have ultrasonography or other supplemental screening. To inform these discussions, this article describes the current state of risk-based breast cancer screening with a focus on breast density. It reviews the evidence regarding its impact relative to other known risk factors for developing breast cancer, and the evidence for and against supplemental screening for women with dense breasts. It also discusses current modalities for supplemental screening beyond mammography, and recommendations for physicians having shared decision-making discussions with women who have dense breasts.

BREAST CANCER RISK FACTORS

The strongest risk factors for breast cancer include age and genetic mutations. Additional known risk factors include breast density, family history, and reproductive history. These risk factors are outlined in **Table 1**, along with their associated relative

Table 1 Relative risks of developing breast cancer for women aged 40 to 49 years	
Risk Factor	**Breast Cancer Risk Ratio (95% CI)**
Two first-degree relatives with breast cancer	3.84 (2.37–6.22)
First-degree relative with breast cancer at age <40 y	3.0 (1.8–4.9)
First-degree relative with breast cancer at age <50 y	2.17 (1.86–2.53)
One first-degree relative with breast cancer	2.14 (1.92–2.38)
Extremely dense breasts on mammography	2.04 (1.84–2.26)
Prior benign breast biopsy	1.87 (1.64–2.13)
Second-degree relative with breast cancer	1.7 (1.4–2.0)
Heterogeneously dense breasts on mammography	1.62 (1.51–1.75)
Current oral contraceptive use	1.30 (1.13–1.49)
Nulliparity	1.25 (1.08–1.46)
Age at first birth ≥30 y	1.20 (1.02–1.42)

Abbreviation: CI, confidence interval.
Adapted from Nelson HD, Zakher B, Cantor A, et al. Risk factors for breast cancer for women age 40 to 49: a systematic review and meta-analysis. Ann Intern Med 2012;156(9):644; with permission.

risks. Factors such as age and genetic mutation status have a larger relative risk than other factors, including breast density.[3]

Even though breast density is a lower risk than other risk factors such as family history, it is more common in the general population. Thus, some researchers have suggested that breast density alone accounts for a considerable proportion of cancer risk at the population level.[3] This finding was supported by Canadian screening program data suggesting that increased breast density accounts for 16% of all breast cancers diagnosed, 40% of interval cancers diagnosed, and 12% of screen-detected cancers.[4]

RISK-BASED SCREENING PROTOCOLS

In the absence of randomized controlled trials evaluating the efficacy of risk-based screening protocols (eg, different intervals or the use of supplemental screening modalities for women at increased risk), simulation modeling studies have provided insight regarding the likely balance between the benefits and risks of different risk-based screening protocols. These modeling studies suggest that screening regimens should be personalized based on a woman's age, breast density, and other risk factors.[5]

One study used several established NCI-funded Cancer Intervention and Surveillance Modeling Network (CISNET) simulation models to determine the most efficient screening strategies based on breast cancer risk. Taking into account advances in imaging and treatment, biennial screening strategies were the most efficient for most women who are at average risk for breast cancer. However, for women with 2-fold to 4-fold increase in risk (eg, family history of breast cancer or extremely dense breasts, defined as those with the highest of 4 categories for breast density, as described later), annual screening beginning at age 40 years had comparable risks and benefits with those of women at average risk undergoing biennial screening between ages 50 and 74 years.[6] Another CISNET study found that women aged 40 to 49 years with a 2-fold increased risk for developing breast cancer (eg, women with extremely dense breasts) have similar harm/benefit risk ratios compared with average-risk women aged 50 to 74 years undergoing biennial screening.[7]

MAMMOGRAPHIC BREAST DENSITY

Given the importance of breast density as a risk factor for breast cancer and increasing attention to screening strategies based on density, a brief background on breast density is provided. Breast density is defined based on a subjective estimate made by an interpreting radiologist of the amount of radiopaque breast parenchyma in relation to radiolucent fatty tissue comprising each breast. This measure does not correlate with physical breast examination findings of breast firmness.[8] In addition, mammographic breast density has been associated with both a masking effect on mammography, in which dense tissue can obscure cancers, as well as an inherent, independent higher risk for the development of breast cancer.[3,4]

According to the American College of Radiology (ACR), breast density should be subjectively classified into 1 of 4 categories by interpreting radiologists under the Breast Imaging Reporting and Data System (BI-RADS): almost entirely fatty, scattered fibroglandular densities, heterogeneously dense, and extremely dense (**Fig. 1**). There is inter-reader and intrareader variability in radiologists' interpretation of breast density. Nevertheless, women who are in the last 2 categories (heterogeneously dense and extremely dense) are commonly grouped together and considered to have dense breasts. About 43% of women aged 40 to 74 years in the United States have heterogeneously or extremely dense breasts by mammography (**Table 2**).

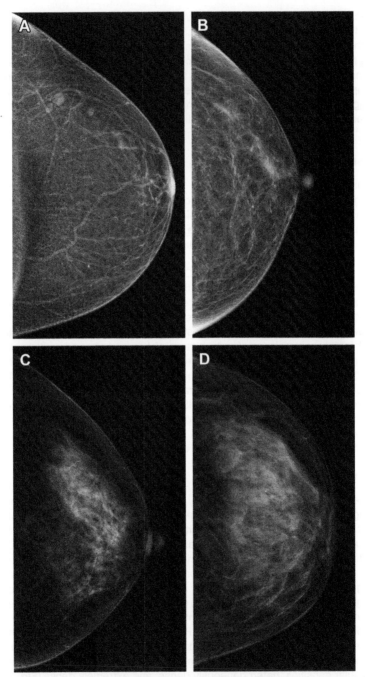

Fig. 1. Density categories by mammography. Multiple craniocaudal views of the left breast in 4 different patients. Approximately 10% of the screening population has almost entirely fatty breasts (*A*), 40% have scattered fibroglandular densities (*B*), 40% have heterogeneously dense breasts (*C*), and 10% have extremely dense breasts (*D*).

Table 2
Density prevalence by age

Age (y)	Distribution of BI-RADS Breast Density Categories (%)			
	Almost Entirely Fatty	Scattered Fibroglandular Densities	Heterogeneously Dense	Extremely Dense
40–44	8	36	44	13
45–49	8	37	43	12
50–54	12	42	38	8
55–59	15	47	33	5
60–64	18	49	29	4
65–69	18	50	28	3
70–74	20	53	24	2
75–79	20	53	25	3
80–84	18	54	26	2
85+	19	54	25	3

Adapted from Sprague BL, Gangnon RE, Trentham-Dietz A, et al. Prevalence of mammographically dense breasts in the United States. J Natl Cancer Inst 2014;106(10):dju255; with permission.

Breast density is influenced by a variety of factors; it usually decreases with increasing age, increases with hormone replacement therapy, and decreases with increasing body mass index. Other modifiable factors influencing breast density include tamoxifen therapy for chemoprevention, and diet changes.[9] Given the moving target of mammographic breast density and its subjective nature, automated software has been developed in an attempt to decrease inter-reader variability, moving toward more quantitative rather than qualitative measures.[10] Although automated quantitative density measurement software is approved by the US Food and Drug Administration (FDA), existing technology is currently limited in accurately estimating three-dimensional (3D) density and is sensitive to breast positioning. Thus, none are currently in wide use for general screening in the United States.[11,12]

BREAST DENSITY AS A DOUBLE-PRONGED RISK

Increased breast density can mask cancers in dense tissue on mammography, leading to lower accuracy of mammography. A study on 329,495 women undergoing screening mammography in the United States between 1996 and 1998 found that mammography had a sensitivity of 87% and specificity of 97% for women with fatty breasts (with 12-month follow-up data to ensure capture of interval cancers). In comparison, sensitivity was 63% and specificity was 89% for women with extremely dense breasts.[13] Mammographic breast density, along with age, remains a primary predictor for the accuracy of screening mammography.[13] Given this, radiologists now frequently reference having heterogeneously or extremely dense breasts as a limitation in their final reports because it decreases the sensitivity of mammography.

The masking effect caused by dense breast tissue has been reduced with the adoption of digital mammography. The Digital Mammographic Imaging Screening Trial (DMIST) showed that the overall diagnostic accuracy of digital mammography is similar to that of screen-film mammography, but that digital mammography is more accurate for women less than age 50 years, women with dense breasts, and women who are premenopausal or perimenopausal.[14] A large prospective cohort study involving more than 300,000 women in the United States found that digital mammography had higher sensitivity for women with extremely dense breasts compared with screen-film mammography (83.6% vs 68.1%; P = .05), confirming DMIST results in US community practice.[15] Digital mammography now comprises more than 95% of mammography units used in the United States and is the standard primary screening modality of choice for women with dense breasts.

Beyond the masking effect, mammographic breast density is also an independent risk factor for the development of breast cancer. It is hypothesized that the greater proportion of epithelial and nonepithelial cells in areas of high breast density, and the greater cumulative exposure to hormones and growth factors, may stimulate more cell division, which increases breast cancer risk.[16] A systematic review and meta-analysis of 42 studies evaluating breast cancer risk related to breast density found that the relative risk of incident breast cancer is 2.92 for women with heterogeneously dense breasts and 4.64 for women with extremely dense breasts compared with women with almost entirely fatty breasts.[17] However, these figures may be misleading because they are comparing relative risks for women with dense breasts with women with almost entirely fatty breasts, which is the lowest classification for breast density and affects only about 10% of the screening population. Instead, compared with women with scattered fibroglandular densities, relative breast cancer risk associated with breast density is much smaller and is estimated to be about 1.2 for women with heterogeneously dense breasts and 2.1 for women with extremely dense breasts.[18] The variable-density comparison groups used in different analyses have led to confusion regarding the true magnitude of cancer risk associated with dense breasts.

Patients have voiced concerns about the increased risk of breast cancer and the potential masking effect on mammography from dense breasts. Fueled by patient advocacy groups, more than half of US states have now adopted legislation requiring radiology facilities to disclose mammography breast density directly to women, many with language recommending that patients discuss options for supplemental screening with their physicians.[19,20] Connecticut was the first state to enact density reporting legislation (in 2011), with some clinicians referring all patients with dense breasts for supplemental ultrasonography in the first year after adoption.[21] National legislation is also currently under consideration, including a proposed amendment to the Public Health Service Act requiring notification of breast density to patients and stating that they may benefit from supplemental screening.[22] With mandatory reporting and greater patient and physician awareness regarding dense breasts, there are increasing opportunities for shared decision making and personalized screening regimens.[23] However, the challenges of classifying density and the limited evidence base need to be considered and are described later.

Tomosynthesis

In 2011, the FDA approved digital breast tomosynthesis for all clinical indications accepted for mammography, including screening. In contrast with digital mammography, tomosynthesis obtains multiple mammographic images with the x-ray source traveling in an arc over the compressed breasts, allowing a 3D reconstruction of the breast.[24] This technology is now a built-in feature of newer-generation digital mammography units and can be obtained during the same compression required for standard digital mammography views. By allowing radiologists to scroll through breasts slice by slice, tomosynthesis can further mitigate the masking effect of dense breasts and allow visualization of small breast cancers.

Early evidence from prospective cohort studies regarding tomosynthesis for population-based screening is limited.[25,26] Interim results from a Norwegian study, involving 12,631 women aged 50 to 69 years, found that adding tomosynthesis to digital mammography screening resulted in a 31% increase in cancer detection rate and a 15% decrease in recall rate.[25] An Italian study showed similar results, with the detection of 8.1 cancers per 1000 screens when tomosynthesis was added, compared with 5.3 cancers per 1000 screens for digital mammography alone, with false-positive recalls decreasing by 17% with the addition of tomosynthesis.[26] The Italian study also showed similar improvements in cancer detection rate beyond digital mammography for women with dense and nondense breasts alike, suggesting that tomosynthesis could be beneficial for all women. However, reports from both European studies were limited by small size and the lack of multiyear follow-up data.

A multicenter, retrospective US cohort study found improvements in cancer detection and recall rates comparable with those of European prospective studies after adoption of tomosynthesis.[27] However, this same study suggested increased breast biopsy rates after tomosynthesis adoption, reflecting the unknown nature of the balance between benefits and harms of tomosynthesis screening. One CISNET modeling study examined the potential of adding tomosynthesis to biennial digital mammography screening for US women aged 50 to 74 years with dense breasts.[28] Researchers found that tomosynthesis screening could avert 0.5 additional breast cancer deaths and 405 false-positive screening examinations among 1000 women screened.[28]

Among most facilities that have adopted tomosynthesis, 3D acquisition is obtained in addition to standard two-dimensional (2D) acquisition. Thus, because 3D acquisition confers a dose comparable with that of standard digital mammography, patients receive about 2 times the usual radiation dose. Increased radiation dose may be mitigated with adoption of FDA-approved software that provides a synthetic 2D mammogram created from 3D acquisition during tomosynthesis, negating the need for both 2D and 3D image acquisition.[29]

Tomosynthesis is increasingly being used in clinical practices in the United States despite this limited evidence base. From 2013 to 2015, tomosynthesis availability in US imaging facilities participating in the Breast Cancer Surveillance Consortium increased from 0% to 50%.[30] Beginning in January 2015, the US Centers for Medicare and Medicaid Services began reimbursing for tomosynthesis for all women regardless of breast density, likely accelerating its rapid adoption. No randomized trial data or long-term follow-up data from any tomosynthesis study are currently available; such studies are necessary to determine the true improvements in accuracy and patient outcomes associated with tomosynthesis.

CHALLENGES OF RISK-BASED SCREENING BASED ON BREAST DENSITY

The classification of women's breast density is complicated by considerable intra-reader and inter-reader variability.[31] Most of the inter-reader agreement is in the 2 classifications at the extreme ends of the spectrum (almost entirely fatty and extremely dense), with considerable variation in agreement between the 2 middle density classes; it is these 2 middle density classes that separate women as having or not having dense breasts according to the US state legislation efforts.[32] In one study of 30 US facilities, assessments of dense breast made by 83 radiologists ranged from 6.3% to 84.5% of all mammograms interpreted by the radiologist, with multivariable adjustments for patient characteristics having little effect on the range of variation.[19] Moreover, from one screening mammogram to the next, 17% of women had discordant assessments with regard to having dense versus nondense breasts, even though breast density likely changes much more gradually and over a longer period of time.[19]

POTENTIAL SUPPLEMENTAL SCREENING MODALITIES FOR WOMEN WITH DENSE BREASTS

Over the last several years, multiple imaging modalities have been proposed as supplemental screening tools for women at increased risk of breast cancer, including women with dense breasts. The potential benefits and harms of different supplemental screening modalities currently available to women with dense breasts are summarized in **Table 3** and described in more detail later.

Ultrasonography

The few states that mandate insurance coverage for supplemental screening require reimbursement for screening ultrasonography.[33] Ultrasonography has the advantage of not emitting ionizing radiation, being well tolerated by patients, and already being widely available at most radiology practices (**Fig. 2**). The disadvantages include the high operator dependence, a slowdown in radiologist workflow, and a lower specificity compared with mammography.

The highest quality data available regarding supplemental ultrasonography for women with dense breasts come from American College of Radiology Imaging

Table 3
Supplemental screening options for women with dense breasts

Imaging Modality	Advantages	Disadvantages
Digital breast tomosynthesis	• Improved cancer detection • Reduced false-positives • Obtained during standard mammogram examination • Widely available • Being adopted as a primary screening modality	• Additional ionizing radiation when added to digital mammography • Additional out-of-pocket costs if payers do not cover it
Screening ultrasonography	• Widely available • Improved cancer detection • No ionizing radiation	• Highly operator dependent • Increased false-positives • Increased benign biopsies • Additional out-of-pocket costs if payers do not cover it
MRI	• Highest sensitivity for detecting additional cancers • No ionizing radiation	• Not widely available • Requires intravenous gadolinium injection • Increased false-positives • Increased benign biopsies • Additional out-of-pocket costs if payers do not cover it
Contrast-enhanced spectral mammography	• Improved cancer detection • Obtained during standard mammogram examination	• Not widely available • Requires intravenous contrast injection • Additional out-of-pocket costs if payers do not cover it • Additional ionizing radiation when added to digital mammography
Molecular breast imaging	• Improved cancer detection • Potentially improved specificity	• Not widely available • Requires intravenous radioactive tracer injection • Additional ionizing radiation

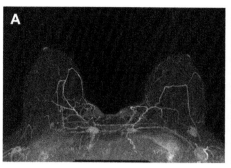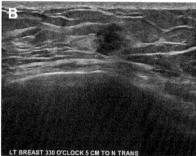

Fig. 2. Supplemental screening breast ultrasonography and MRI. (*A*) A maximum intensity projection image from a screening MRI scan showing a suspicious mass in the left breast that was subsequently biopsied and found to be early-stage invasive ductal carcinoma. (*B*) Handheld screening ultrasonography of the left breast with an irregular hypoechoic mass identified and found to be early-stage invasive ductal carcinoma after ultrasonography-guided biopsy.

Network (ACRIN) 6666, a study of US women with heterogeneously or extremely dense breasts and at least 1 other risk factor (eg, family history). This large, prospective, multi-institutional trial showed that supplemental ultrasonography screening led to incremental cancer detection increases of 3 to 4 per 1000.[34] Most of these additional cancer cases were early invasive cancers with a lower stage and higher likelihood of survival. However, adding ultrasonography after a negative mammogram also increased false-positives and benign biopsies, and decreased overall screening positive predictive value (PPV).[34] A recent systematic review conducted for the USPSTF found that ultrasonography after a negative mammogram had a sensitivity of 80% to 83%, specificity of 86% to 95%, and PPV of 3% to 8%.[35] Real-world data regarding supplemental ultrasonography for women with dense breasts suggest that the incremental cancer detection rate is less than that seen in ACRIN 6666.[36]

Several CISNET models were used to evaluate supplemental screening ultrasonography after negative mammography for women with dense breasts aged 50 to 74 years.[37] In a comparative modeling study, researchers found that adding ultrasonography averted 0.36 additional breast cancer deaths but resulted in 354 unnecessary benign biopsies per 1000 women screened.[37] Even though the comparative weighting of rare benefits of deaths prevented and more common risks such as benign biopsies is subjective, researchers concluded that adding ultrasonography to digital mammography screening likely causes more harm relative to benefits gained.

Handheld ultrasonography examinations have the disadvantage of being highly operator dependent. To offer reduced operator dependence, automated whole-breast ultrasonography (ABUS) was approved as a new screening modality by the FDA in 2012. ABUS involves automated sweeps through the entirety of both breasts and can be administered by technologists. Early studies show promise for ABUS for detecting additional cancers.[38–40] However, its limitations include high false-positive rates, the need to obtain additional handheld ultrasonography data for indeterminate findings, and radiologists' interpretive time for reviewing the hundreds of images obtained.[41]

MRI

MRI is considered the most sensitive imaging modality for detecting breast cancer (see **Fig. 2**), but has low specificity, requires intravenous gadolinium injection, and is associated with a higher false-positive rate and higher costs. The American Cancer Society and other medical societies consider MRI an effective adjunct screening tool for *BRCA* mutation carriers and other women with greater than 20% lifetime risk of developing breast cancer[42]; however, these recommendations are based on added incidence risk, rather than added mortality risk. Moreover, there is little evidence to support MRI for women with dense breasts and no other risk factors. A systematic review found that, among women with dense breasts, MRI has a sensitivity of 75% to 100%, specificity of 78% to 94%, and a PPV of 3% to 33%.[35] When added to mammography screening for women with dense breasts, MRI detects 3.5 to 28.6 additional cancers per 1000 women, but is associated with a recall rate of 12% to 24%.[35]

A subset of patients in ACRIN 6666, with breast density and at least 1 other risk factor (thus, intermediate risk), had an additional MRI added to mammography and ultrasonography screening. This subanalysis showed that women who had supplemental MRI had a higher cancer yield and lower false-positive rate than women who had supplemental ultrasonography.[43] Thus, for women who have dense breasts and other risk factors that push them over the greater than 20% lifetime risk threshold, supplemental MRI is preferred to ultrasonography. To address the lengthy MRI protocol that decreases the level of patient tolerance (30–45 minutes in length), fast MRI is currently being developed. This abbreviated protocol takes about 3 minutes to acquire images. In early studies for screening women with dense breasts and negative screening mammograms and ultrasonography scans, fast MRI has been associated with negative predictive value of 99.8% and a cancer detection rate of 18.3 per 1000 women.[44]

Alternative Functional Imaging

MRI is more effective than ultrasonography for detecting breast cancers because its interpretation is not hindered by breast density and it provides more functional information for breast masses, including lesion vascularity. Dual-energy contrast-enhanced spectral mammography takes advantage of widely available iodinated contrast to detect enhancing lesions within the breast by comparing precontrast and postcontrast mammography images. Early studies suggest that this technique is faster and cheaper than MRI, and that it has the ability to detect nearly all invasive cancers with fewer false-positives than MRI.[45] Similarly, nuclear medicine techniques can provide information about metabolic activity that is more suggestive of breast cancers using available radiotracers and are effective in cancer detection independent of breast density.[46] Newer breast-specific gamma cameras can achieve improved spatial resolution, allowing improved detection of smaller invasive cancers and acquisition of images in projections mimicking those of a standard mammogram.[47,48]

Molecular breast imaging (MBI) techniques, which use intravenous technetium 99m–sestamibi, are not currently in widespread use. Early studies suggest increased sensitivity and an improved PPV for MBI plus mammography, versus mammography alone, among women with dense breasts.[47,48] However, the additional systemic radiation dose from MBI poses an increased lifetime radiation-induced cancer risk if used repeatedly as an adjunct screening tool. In addition, MBI requires nearby production and storage of radioactive tracers, limiting patient access.

NATIONAL GROUP RECOMMENDATIONS

Most national groups agree that the primary screening modality for women with dense breasts is routine digital mammography (**Table 4**). Even though early studies on tomosynthesis are promising, most authoritative bodies claim that there is insufficient

Table 4
Current national group positions on screening women with dense breasts

National Group	Year	Recommendation Statement on Primary Screening	Recommendation Statement on Supplemental Screening
USPSTF[1,2]	2009/2016	"For younger women and women with dense breast tissue, overall detection is somewhat better with digital mammography (2009)"	"[T]he current evidence is insufficient to assess the balance of benefits and harms of adjunctive screening for breast cancer using breast ultrasonography, MRI, DBT [digital breast tomosynthesis], or other methods in women identified to have dense breasts on an otherwise negative screening mammogram (2016)"
ACS[2]	2015	"Although overall the sensitivity of digital and screen-film mammography is similar, digital mammography is more sensitive in younger women and women with mammographically dense breasts"	"Accumulating data on digital breast tomosynthesis (DBT) appear to demonstrate further improvements in accuracy (both sensitivity and specificity), and DBT is steadily increasing in prevalence in mammography facilities." "The [guideline development group] also did not include in this review evidence on the effectiveness of supplemental breast imaging for women with mammographically dense breasts"
ACR[60]	2013	Annual screening mammography is indicated for high-risk and intermediate-risk women. In addition, for high-risk women, contrast-enhanced MRI is indicated. Ultrasonography can be considered as an alternative for those with contraindications to MRI	"[M]ammography alone does not perform as well as mammography plus supplemental screening in certain subsets of women, particularly those with genetic predispositions to the disease and those with dense breasts" "Supplemental screening with ultrasound for women with intermediate risk and dense breasts is an option to increase cancer detection"
NCCN[61]	2016	"Digital mammography appears to benefit young women and women with dense breasts"	"Although there are some studies supporting the use of ultrasound for breast cancer screening as an adjunct to mammography for high risk women with dense breast tissue, the NCCN Panel however cautions that there is insufficient evidence to support routine supplemental screening in women with dense breasts and no other risk factors"

Abbreviation: NCCN, National Comprehensive Cancer Network.

evidence to recommend routine tomosynthesis screening.[1] The American College of Physicians goes a step further and currently advises against screening women at average risk for breast cancer with tomosynthesis, citing a current lack of evidence for improved value in care.[49]

Moreover, no supplemental screening modalities are currently recommended for women with dense breasts by most national organizations (see **Table 4**).[1,50] At present, only the ACR considers supplemental ultrasonography an appropriate supplemental screening option for women who have dense breasts and at least 1 additional risk factor.[51] Even though supplemental screening ultrasonography is covered by insurance in a few US states because of mandatory density reporting laws, there is currently no evidence to support routine use of supplemental screening ultrasonography in patients with dense breasts and no other risk factors.[52] There are currently several ongoing large-scale trials designed to address the efficacy of multi-modality screening for women with dense breasts.[53,54]

SHARED DECISION-MAKING DISCUSSIONS

At present, more than half of the US states have implemented some sort of breast density notification law. In response to this legislation, and the likely increase in patient awareness and inquiry around supplemental screening, several efforts have taken place to help provide guidance for shared decision-making conversations between primary care physicians and their patients. Clear communication between physicians and women with dense breasts following these mandatory notifications is especially critical given that the wording used in the dense breast notifications scores low on readability and understandability, meaning that these reports are likely difficult for women to interpret.[55] Several recommendations for physicians engaging in these discussions are outlined later.

First, physicians must understand the patient's risk profile. Although breast density is an independent risk factor for the development of breast cancer, the actual risk of developing breast cancer when high breast density is the patient's only risk factor is low (**Table 5**).[56] In addition, the current evidence suggests that breast density should not be the sole factor for pursuing supplemental screening. This suggestion has been supported by a recent prospective cohort study from the United States that found that

Table 5				
Absolute 5-year risk of breast cancer by age and density				
	5-y Risk for Breast Cancer by Density (%)			
Age (y)	**Almost Entirely Fatty**	**Scattered Fibroglandular Densities**	**Heterogeneously Dense**	**Extremely Dense**
40–44	0.2	0.5	0.7	1.0
45–49	0.4	0.8	1.2	1.6
50–54	0.5	1.0	1.6	2.1
55–59	0.7	1.4	2.2	3.0
60–64	0.8	1.7	2.6	3.4
65–69	1.3	2.0	2.9	3.0
70–74	1.4	2.1	3.1	3.3

Adapted from Tice JA, Cummings SR, Smith-Bindman R, et al. Using clinical factors and mammographic breast density to estimate breast cancer risk: development and validation of a new predictive model. Ann Intern Med 2008;148(5):343; with permission.

not all women with dense breasts have high interval cancer rates.[57] Researchers found that 5-year cancer risk was low to average for 51.0% of women with heterogeneously dense breasts and 52.5% of women with extremely dense breasts in a cohort of 365,426 women aged 40 to 74 years. Thus, women whose only risk factor is high breast density are unlikely to benefit from supplemental screening.

Second, in order to determine a woman's overall risk profile, physicians should use an established risk model or calculator. Models such as BRCAPRO, Tyrer-Cuzick, and Claus offer estimates of lifetime risk, whereas the Breast Cancer Surveillance Consortium (BCSC) risk calculator offers estimates of risk for the next 5 and 10 years. It is important that formal risk assessment should take all of a patient's risk factors into account when determining a personalized screening approach. Online and easily accessible risk assessment tools include the National Cancer Institute's Breast Cancer Risk Assessment Tool (https://www.cancer.gov/bcrisktool/) and the BCSC Risk Calculator (https://tools.bcsc-scc.org/bc5yearrisk/calculator.htm). Only the latter incorporates the woman's mammographic breast density into its risk calculations.

For women at average risk (ie, lifetime risk <15%), regardless of breast density, no supplemental screening beyond digital mammography is recommended. For women at high risk (ie, lifetime risk >20%), regardless of breast density, supplemental screening is recommended in the form of breast MRI.[58] The addition of supplemental ultrasonography is unnecessary for these patients because a large multi-institutional trial showed that no additional cancers were detected with ultrasonography beyond those found by mammography and MRI.[43] For women with dense breasts and intermediate risk (ie, 15%–20% lifetime risk), a discussion about the supplemental screening options, such as screening ultrasonography, and their associated benefits and risks is suggested. For women at intermediate to high risk, shared decision-making conversations about screening can also involve discussion about potential risk-reducing therapies, such as tamoxifen.

These shared decision-making conversations should cover risks, benefits, alternatives, and patient preferences regarding supplemental screening. A Cochrane Review of trials examining personalized risk communication on informed decision making suggested that such communications related to breast cancer screening led to increased knowledge and accuracy in personal risk perception among patients.[59] Although physicians can serve as experts regarding the clinical evidence, the eventual choice for supplemental screening should be based on the patient's values. For those women at low or average risk who choose supplemental screening for dense breasts against clinical recommendations, ultrasonography is the cheaper and more accessible option. Patients should be warned that, except for a few US states that have mandated insurance coverage for additional supplemental screening, most women incur additional out-of-pocket expenses to undergo supplemental screening.

SUMMARY

Fueled by patient advocacy groups, there is growing interest in better understanding the increased cancer risk and decreased mammography accuracy associated with breast density. Compared with screen-film mammography, digital mammography shows higher accuracy for screening women with dense breasts and represents the primary screening modality of choice. Digital breast tomosynthesis, or 3D mammography, shows early promise for mitigating the masking effect of dense breast tissue, although evidence regarding the effectiveness of tomosynthesis is lacking. Screening ultrasonography likely improves cancer detection but also increases recall and biopsy rates. While awaiting results from ongoing trials that will help women with dense breasts decide on the most appropriate multimodality screening regimens, physicians should be able to understand and communicate the absolute and relative risk of dense breasts and review the available options with patients. In addition, physicians should remember to consider breast density as only 1 factor when determining risk-based screening approaches for individual women.

REFERENCES

1. Siu AL, Force US Preventive Services Task Force. Screening for Breast Cancer: U.S. Preventive Services Task Force recommendation statement. Ann Intern Med 2016;164(4):279–96.
2. Oeffinger KC, Fontham ET, Etzioni R, et al. Breast cancer screening for women at average risk: 2015 guideline update from the American Cancer Society. JAMA 2015;314(15):1599–614.
3. Boyd NF, Martin LJ, Yaffe MJ, et al. Mammographic density and breast cancer risk: current understanding and future prospects. Breast Cancer Res 2011; 13(6):223.
4. Boyd NF, Guo H, Martin LJ, et al. Mammographic density and the risk and detection of breast cancer. N Engl J Med 2007;356(3):227–36.
5. Schousboe JT, Kerlikowske K, Loh A, et al. Personalizing mammography by breast density and other risk factors for breast cancer: analysis of health benefits and cost-effectiveness. Ann Intern Med 2011;155(1):10–20.
6. Mandelblatt JS, Stout NK, Schechter CB, et al. Collaborative modeling of the benefits and harms associated with different U.S. breast cancer screening strategies. Ann Intern Med 2016;164(4):215–25.
7. van Ravesteyn NT, Miglioretti DL, Stout NK, et al. Tipping the balance of benefits and harms to favor screening mammography starting at age 40 years: a comparative modeling study of risk. Ann Intern Med 2012;156(9):609–17.
8. Swann CA, Kopans DB, McCarthy KA, et al. Mammographic density and physical assessment of the breast. AJR Am J Roentgenol 1987;148(3):525–6.
9. Vachon CM, Kushi LH, Cerhan JR, et al. Association of diet and mammographic breast density in the Minnesota Breast Cancer Family Cohort. Cancer Epidemiol Biomarkers Prev 2000;9(2):151–60.
10. Spayne MC, Gard CC, Skelly J, et al. Reproducibility of BI-RADS breast density measures among community radiologists: a prospective cohort study. Breast J 2012;18(4):326–33.
11. Ciatto S, Bernardi D, Calabrese M, et al. A first evaluation of breast radiological density assessment by QUANTRA software as compared to visual classification. Breast 2012;21(4):503–6.
12. Alonzo-Proulx O, Jong RA, Yaffe MJ. Volumetric breast density characteristics as determined from digital mammograms. Phys Med Biol 2012;57(22):7443–57.
13. Carney PA, Miglioretti DL, Yankaskas BC, et al. Individual and combined effects of age, breast density, and hormone replacement therapy use on the accuracy of screening mammography. Ann Intern Med 2003;138(3):168–75.
14. Pisano ED, Gatsonis C, Hendrick E, et al. Diagnostic performance of digital versus film mammography for breast-cancer screening. N Engl J Med 2005; 353(17):1773–83.
15. Kerlikowske K, Hubbard RA, Miglioretti DL, et al. Comparative effectiveness of digital versus film-screen mammography in community practice in the United States: a cohort study. Ann Intern Med 2011;155(8):493–502.

16. Kerlikowske K, Ichikawa L, Miglioretti DL, et al. Longitudinal measurement of clinical mammographic breast density to improve estimation of breast cancer risk. J Natl Cancer Inst 2007;99(5):386–95.

17. McCormack VA, dos Santos Silva I. Breast density and parenchymal patterns as markers of breast cancer risk: a meta-analysis. Cancer Epidemiol Biomarkers Prev 2006;15(6):1159–69.

18. Sickles EA. The use of breast imaging to screen women at high risk for cancer. Radiol Clin North Am 2010;48(5):859–78.

19. Sprague BL, Conant EF, Onega T, et al. Variation in mammographic breast density assessments among radiologists in clinical practice: a multicenter observational study. Ann Intern Med 2016;165(7):457–64.

20. Lee CI, Lehman CD. Digital breast tomosynthesis and the challenges of implementing an emerging breast cancer screening technology into clinical practice. J Am Coll Radiol 2013;10(12):913–7.

21. Hooley RJ, Greenberg KL, Stackhouse RM, et al. Screening US in patients with mammographically dense breasts: initial experience with Connecticut Public Act 09-41. Radiology 2012;265(1):59–69.

22. Freer PE. Mammographic breast density: impact on breast cancer risk and implications for screening. Radiographics 2015;35(2):302–15.

23. Lee CI, Bassett LW, Lehman CD. Breast density legislation and opportunities for patient-centered outcomes research. Radiology 2012;264(3):632–6.

24. Baker JA, Lo JY. Breast tomosynthesis: state-of-the-art and review of the literature. Acad Radiol 2011;18(10):1298–310.

25. Skaane P, Bandos AI, Gullien R, et al. Comparison of digital mammography alone and digital mammography plus tomosynthesis in a population-based screening program. Radiology 2013;267(1):47–56.

26. Ciatto S, Houssami N, Bernardi D, et al. Integration of 3D digital mammography with tomosynthesis for population breast-cancer screening (STORM): a prospective comparison study. Lancet Oncol 2013;14(7):583–9.

27. Friedewald SM, Rafferty EA, Rose SL, et al. Breast cancer screening using tomosynthesis in combination with digital mammography. JAMA 2014;311(24):2499–507.

28. Lee CI, Cevik M, Alagoz O, et al. Comparative effectiveness of combined digital mammography and tomosynthesis screening for women with dense breasts. Radiology 2015;274(3):772–80.

29. Zuley ML, Guo B, Catullo VJ, et al. Comparison of two-dimensional synthesized mammograms versus original digital mammograms alone and in combination with tomosynthesis images. Radiology 2014;271(3):664–71.

30. Houssami N, Miglioretti DL. Digital breast tomosynthesis: a brave new world of mammography screening. JAMA Oncol 2016;2(6):725–7.

31. Kerlikowske K, Grady D, Barclay J, et al. Variability and accuracy in mammographic interpretation using the American College of Radiology Breast Imaging Reporting and Data System. J Natl Cancer Inst 1998;90(23):1801–9.

32. Nicholson BT, LoRusso AP, Smolkin M, et al. Accuracy of assigned BI-RADS breast density category definitions. Acad Radiol 2006;13(9):1143–9.

33. Dehkordy SF, Carlos RC. Dense breast legislation in the United States: state of the states. J Am Coll Radiol 2013;10(12):899–902.

34. Berg WA, Blume JD, Cormack JB, et al. Combined screening with ultrasound and mammography vs mammography alone in women at elevated risk of breast cancer. JAMA 2008;299(18):2151–63.

35. Melnikow J, Fenton JJ, Whitlock EP, et al. Supplemental screening for breast cancer in women with dense breasts: a systematic review for the U.S. Preventive Services Task Force. Ann Intern Med 2016;164(4):268–78.

36. Parris T, Wakefield D, Frimmer H. Real world performance of screening breast ultrasound following enactment of Connecticut Bill 458. Breast J 2013;19(1):64–70.

37. Sprague BL, Stout NK, Schechter C, et al. Benefits, harms, and cost-effectiveness of supplemental ultrasonography screening for women with dense breasts. Ann Intern Med 2015;162(3):157–66.

38. Kelly KM, Dean J, Comulada WS, et al. Breast cancer detection using automated whole breast ultrasound and mammography in radiographically dense breasts. Eur Radiol 2010;20(3):734–42.

39. Kelly KM, Dean J, Lee SJ, et al. Breast cancer detection: radiologists' performance using mammography with and without automated whole-breast ultrasound. Eur Radiol 2010;20(11):2557–64.

40. Giuliano V, Giuliano C. Improved breast cancer detection in asymptomatic women using 3D-automated breast ultrasound in mammographically dense breasts. Clin Imaging 2013;37(3):480–6.

41. Chang JM, Moon WK, Cho N, et al. Breast cancers initially detected by hand-held ultrasound: detection performance of radiologists using automated breast ultrasound data. Acta Radiol 2011;52(1):8–14.

42. Saslow D, Boetes C, Burke W, et al. American Cancer Society guidelines for breast screening with MRI as an adjunct to mammography. CA Cancer J Clin 2007;57(2):75–89.

43. Berg WA, Zhang Z, Lehrer D, et al. Detection of breast cancer with addition of annual screening ultrasound or a single screening MRI to mammography in women with elevated breast cancer risk. JAMA 2012;307(13):1394–404.

44. Kuhl CK, Schrading S, Strobel K, et al. Abbreviated breast magnetic resonance imaging (MRI): first postcontrast subtracted images and maximum-intensity projection-a novel approach to breast cancer screening with MRI. J Clin Oncol 2014; 32(22):2304–10.

45. Jochelson MS, Dershaw DD, Sung JS, et al. Bilateral contrast-enhanced dual-energy digital mammography: feasibility and comparison with conventional digital mammography and MR imaging in women with known breast carcinoma. Radiology 2013;266(3):743–51.

46. Khalkhali I, Baum JK, Villanueva-Meyer J, et al. (99m)Tc sestamibi breast imaging for the examination of patients with dense and fatty breasts: multicenter study. Radiology 2002;222(1):149–55.

47. Brem RF, Floerke AC, Rapelyea JA, et al. Breast-specific gamma imaging as an adjunct imaging modality for the diagnosis of breast cancer. Radiology 2008; 247(3):651–7.

48. Rhodes DJ, Hruska CB, Phillips SW, et al. Dedicated dual-head gamma imaging for breast cancer screening in women with mammographically dense breasts. Radiology 2011;258(1):106–18.

49. Wilt TJ, Harris RP, Qaseem A, High Value Care Task Force of the American College of Physicians. Screening for cancer: advice for high-value care from the American College of Physicians. Ann Intern Med 2015;162(10):718–25.

50. Bevers T, Bibbins-Domingo K, Oeffinger KC, et al. Controversies in breast cancer screening strategies. J Natl Compr Canc Netw 2016;14(5 Suppl):651–3.

51. Mainiero MB, Lourenco A, Mahoney MC, et al. ACR appropriateness criteria breast cancer screening. J Am Coll Radiol 2013;10(1):11–4.

52. Gartlehner G, Thaler K, Chapman A, et al. Mammography in combination with breast ultrasonography versus mammography for breast cancer screening in women at average risk. Cochrane Database Syst Rev 2013;(4):CD009632.

53. Tagliafico AS, Calabrese M, Mariscotti G, et al. Adjunct screening with tomosynthesis or ultrasound in women with mammography-negative dense breasts: interim report of a prospective comparative trial. J Clin Oncol 2016. [Epub ahead of print].

54. Emaus MJ, Bakker MF, Peeters PH, et al. MR imaging as an additional screening modality for the detection of breast cancer in women aged 50-75 years with extremely dense breasts: The DENSE Trial Study Design. Radiology 2015; 277(2):527–37.

55. Kressin NR, Gunn CM, Battaglia TA. Content, readability, and understandability of dense breast notifications by state. JAMA 2016;315(16):1786–8.

56. Tice JA, Cummings SR, Smith-Bindman R, et al. Using clinical factors and mammographic breast density to estimate breast cancer risk: development and validation of a new predictive model. Ann Intern Med 2008;148(5):337–47.

57. Kerlikowske K, Zhu W, Tosteson AN, et al. Identifying women with dense breasts at high risk for interval cancer: a cohort study. Ann Intern Med 2015;162(10): 673–81.

58. Freer PE, Slanetz PJ, Haas JS, et al. Breast cancer screening in the era of density notification legislation: summary of 2014 Massachusetts experience and suggestion of an evidence-based management algorithm by multi-disciplinary expert panel. Breast Cancer Res Treat 2015;153(2):455–64.

59. Edwards AG, Naik G, Ahmed H, et al. Personalised risk communication for informed decision making about taking screening tests. Cochrane Database Syst Rev 2013;(2):CD001865.

60. Lee CH, Dershaw DD, Kopans D, et al. Breast cancer screening with imaging: recommendations from the Society of Breast Imaging and the ACR on the use of mammography, breast MRI, breast ultrasound, and other technologies for the detection of clinically occult breast cancer. J Am Coll Radiol 2010;7(1):18–27.

61. National Comprehensive Cancer Network. Breast Cancer Screening and Diagnosis. Available at: https://www.nccn.org/professionals/physician_gls/f_guidelines.asp#detection. Accessed November 22, 2016.

Cervical Cancer Screening

George F. Sawaya, MD[a,b,*], Megan J. Huchko, MD, MPH[c]

KEYWORDS

- Cervical cancer screening • Cervical cancer prevention
- Human papillomavirus vaccination • Human papillomavirus testing
- Cervical cytology • High-value care • Preterm birth

KEY POINTS

- Cervical cancer screening in the United States has accompanied profound decreases in cancer incidence and mortality over the last half century.
- Current screening guidelines issued by major groups are largely consistent and strive to find a reasonable balance between benefits and harms by recommending less screening in most women.
- Two strategies are endorsed by major US-based guideline groups: (1) triennial cytology for women aged 21 to 65 years, and (2) triennial cytology for women aged 21 to 29 years followed by cytology plus testing for high-risk human papillomavirus types every 5 years for women aged 30 years and older.
- Maintaining gains in cervical cancer prevention requires a continued vigilant approach that includes access to low-cost, high-quality screening for all women and appropriate human papilloma virus vaccination.
- As new screening strategies emerge and are adopted, comparative effectiveness analyses will be needed to outline the patient-centered and economic implications of choosing one rather than another.

Disclosure: Dr G.F. Sawaya is funded by NIH (1R01CA169093) to identify the range of reasonable options for cervical cancer screening from a patient-centered and economic perspective. Dr M. J. Huchko is funded by NIH (5R01CA188248 and U54CA190153) to evaluate implementation strategies for cervical screening programs in low-resource settings. The authors declare no commercial or other financial conflicts of interest.

[a] Department of Obstetrics, Gynecology and Reproductive Sciences, University of California, San Francisco, 550 16th Street, Floor 7, San Francisco, CA 94143, USA; [b] Department of Epidemiology & Biostatistics, University of California, San Francisco, 550 16th Street, Floor 7, San Francisco, CA 94143, USA; [c] Department of Obstetrics and Gynecology, Global Health Institute, Duke University, 310 Trent Drive, Box 90519, Durham, NC, 27708, USA
* Corresponding author. Department of Obstetrics, Gynecology and Reproductive Sciences, University of California, San Francisco, 550 16th Street, Floor 7, San Francisco, CA 94143.
E-mail address: george.sawaya@ucsf.edu

Med Clin N Am 101 (2017) 743–753
http://dx.doi.org/10.1016/j.mcna.2017.03.006
0025-7125/17/© 2017 Elsevier Inc. All rights reserved.

INTRODUCTION

Cervical cancer is an uncommon disease in the United States, with an estimated 13,000 incident cases and 4100 deaths occurring in 2016.[1] Rates have steadily declined over the last few decades coincident with widespread, population-based screening. Disparities in incidence and mortality are still noted, with black and Hispanic women continuing to have higher rates of cervical cancer than white women.

High-quality evidence implicates high-risk human papillomavirus (HPV) types as the causative agents in cervical cancer. HPV infections are common; the US Centers for Disease Control and Prevention (CDC) estimates that nearly all sexually active women are exposed to HPV over their lifetimes.[2] Although most infections resolve without consequence, persistent infections can lead to precancerous cervical lesions and, in a minority of women, invasive cancer.

The most common precancerous lesions are of squamous cell origin, called cervical intraepithelial neoplasia (CIN), and are graded by the proportion of abnormal epithelium.

- CIN grade 1 indicates an active HPV infection and these lesions are considered low grade with a high spontaneous regression rate; these lesions are generally not treated.
- CIN grade 2 is often considered a high-grade lesion but has a spontaneous regression rate of up to 40%.
- CIN grade 3 lesions have the highest likelihood of progression to invasion and are universally treated.

The estimated time for CIN grade 3 progression to cancer is on average 10 years, allowing many opportunities for these lesions to be found and treated. Preinvasive lesions of glandular cell origin (adenocarcinoma in situ) are less common but are of such concern that hysterectomy is recommended when diagnosed. Of note, cytology-based screening has led to declines in the incidence and mortality of squamous cell cancer but not in cancers of glandular origin.

High-grade CIN lesions (CIN2 and CIN3) are treated with either ablation (eg, laser, cryotherapy) or excision (eg, loop excision, cone biopsy).[3] Both treatments have high efficacy (short-term cure rates of 85%–95%) but have different side effects. The association between excisional procedures and preterm birth has led to a more cautious use of these techniques. Prior systematic reviews have found no associations between cryotherapy and laser ablation and preterm birth.[4] More recent reviews have noted increases in the risk of preterm birth as excision depths increase as well as small increases with unspecified ablative treatments.[5] As with much evidence about harm, the observational nature of current studies limits causal inference; the relationship between cervical treatments and preterm birth may be confounded by a third factor affecting risk of both. Acknowledging these potential harms, treatment guidelines by the American Congress of Obstetricians and Gynecologists (ACOG) suggest a judicious approach when treatment is warranted; for example, the guidelines encourage surveillance of CIN2 rather than treatment, especially in young women.[6]

Three highly effective HPV vaccines have been developed to target up to 9 HPV subtypes, covering either the most common oncogenic types (bivalent vaccine against 16/18), or a combination of these plus the condyloma-causing HPV types 6 and 11 (quadrivalent vaccine, now replaced by a nonavalent vaccine). Targeted to adolescents of both sexes, the vaccines have been shown to decrease the incidence of both HPV and CIN, with rates of up to 100% efficacy against the vaccine-specific HPV types and related disease in women who have not been previously exposed.[7,8] HPV vaccines show little cross-protection against other oncogenic subtypes, and effectiveness decreases when administered to older women and women who have previously been exposed to HPV.[9] Therefore, although the overall population effectiveness is likely to be lower than the efficacy seen in the clinical trials, widespread vaccine uptake is anticipated to result in a decrease in CIN and cervical cancer in the future and may affect the design of screening and treatment programs.[10,11]

SCREENING PROGRAMS IN THE UNITED STATES

About 90% of US women report having had screening within the prior 5 years, which is a testament to the acceptability of speculum examinations for collection of cervical specimens.[12] With screening, it is estimated that the lifetime risk of being diagnosed with cervical cancer in the United States is 0.6%.[1] Among women developing cancer, 50% to 60% have never been screened or not adequately screened, emphasizing the importance of finding innovative ways to provide access to high-quality, low-cost screening to women not engaged in screening programs.[13]

As with many cancers, the benefits of cervical cancer screening are well known: decreasing cancer incidence and mortality and perhaps decreasing morbidity to some degree by finding early-stage cancers that are treated with less morbid therapies than those recommended to women with late-stage cancers. In addition, like most cancers, the harms of screening are difficult to measure and often underestimated. For cervical cancer screening, these include false-positive testing, invasive procedures and treatments, psychological distress, and extended surveillance of unclear end. From a societal perspective, costs of various screening strategies need to be understood to ensure that care meets a standard of being high-value.[14]

Cytology-based screening has been the typical approach for decades and has evidence of high effectiveness, but it has been criticized for having a low sensitivity in the detection of high-grade CIN in a single episode of screening. In addition, some common cytologic interpretations (eg, atypical squamous cells of undetermined significance [ASC-US]) have low specificity and positive predictive value. In addition, cytology results lack objectivity, leading to high interobserver variations. In one large US study, agreement between community reading and expert reviews were only moderate for cytologic interpretations (kappa, 0.46; 95% confidence interval, 0.44–0.48).[15]

The introduction of reliable, reproducible tests for the detection of 13 or 14 HPV types implicated in cervical cancer (high-risk HPV [hrHPV]) has expanded options for screening. Summary evidence indicates that hrHPV testing has a higher sensitivity than cytology in detecting high-grade CIN[16] and can be useful in increasing the specificity of some test interpretations (eg, ASC-US).[17]

CURRENT SCREENING STRATEGIES: AVERAGE-RISK WOMEN

In 2012, ACOG,[18] the US Preventive Services Task Force (USPSTF),[19] and the American Cancer Society (ACS) in collaboration with the American Society of Colposcopy and Cervical Cytology (ASCCP) and the American Society of Clinical Pathologists (ASCP)[20] published similar screening guidelines; ACOG updated its guidelines in 2016[6] (**Table 1**). The guidelines focus on average-risk women, defined as women with no prior diagnosis of CIN2 or a more severe lesion or cervical cancer (CIN2+), women who are not immunocompromised (eg, infected with human immunodeficiency virus [HIV]), and women with no in utero exposure to diethylstilbestrol.

All guidelines agree that screening should not begin before age 21 years, regardless of sexual history, and that it be performed no more often than every 3 years. Decision

Table 1
Current recommendations for cervical cancer screening by the US Preventive Services Task Force (2012), American Cancer Society[a] (2012), and/or American Congress of Obstetricians and Gynecologists (2016)

Average-risk Women[b]	
Age to begin	21 y
Method and intervals, by age	Ages 21–65 y: cytology every 3 y Or Ages 21–29 y: cytology every 3 y, then Ages 30–65 y: cytology plus hrHPV testing every 5 y
Age to end	65 y[c]
Higher-risk Women (ACOG 2016)	
Infected with HIV	Age to begin: initiation of sexual activity, but no later than age 21 y Ages 21–29 y: cytology every year until 3 normal tests, then every 3 y Ages 30–65 y: cytology every year until 3 normal tests, then every 3 y, or: cytology plus hrHPV testing every 3 y Age to end: none
Immunocompromised for non-HIV reasons	Screening beginning at age 21 y, then as for women infected with HIV
In utero exposure to diethylstilbestrol	Annual cytology screening
Low-risk Women (ACOG 2016)	
After total hysterectomy, no prior CIN2+	Screening should not be performed

Abbreviation: HIV, human immunodeficiency virus.
[a] With the American Society of Colposcopy and Cervical Pathology and the American Society of Clinical Pathologists.
[b] Recommendations apply to women with no prior diagnosis of CIN2 or a more severe lesion or cervical cancer (CIN2+), women who are not immunocompromised (eg, HIV infected) and women with no in utero exposure to diethylstilbestrol.
[c] Only among women with 3 consecutive negative cytology results or 2 consecutive negative cytology plus hrHPV tests within 10 years before cessation of screening, with the most recent test performed within the last 5 years.

analyses commissioned by the USPSTF indicated that screening more frequently than every 3 years confers small additional reductions in cancer risk, but incurs substantially more screening harms, including false-positive testing and colposcopies.[21] To mitigate harms, ACOG and ACS/ASCCP/ASCP guidelines specifically discourage annual screening among average-risk women of any age. For women aged 30 years and older, the addition of hrHPV testing to cytology allows the stratification of women with normal cytology and negative HPV tests into a particularly low-risk group in which the frequency of screening can be extended to 5 years, and for identifying women with mild cytologic changes (eg, ASC-US) whose underlying risk of CIN2+ is high enough to refer to colposcopy when HPV testing is positive.

All guidelines agree that screening can end at age 65 years of age if the following criteria are met: 3 consecutive negative cytology results or 2 consecutive negative cytology plus hrHPV tests within 10 years before cessation of screening, with the most recent test performed within the last 5 years. The ACS/ASCCP/ASCP guidelines state that once screening has been discontinued, it should not be restarted, regardless of the acquisition of new sexual partners.

CURRENT SCREENING STRATEGIES: HIGHER-RISK WOMEN

Guidelines exclude women at higher than average risk: immune-compromised women, those with prior high-grade CIN or cancer, and those with in utero exposure to diethylstilbestrol. The Panel on Opportunistic Infections in HIV-Infected Adults and Adolescents recommends beginning screening women infected with HIV at the onset of sexual activity and no later than age 21 years, and continuing over a lifetime (not ending at 65 years of age).[22] The panel suggests annual screening with cytology alone or cytology plus hrHPV testing for women aged 30 years and older. Intervals can be lengthened to 3 years among those with 3 prior normal cytology tests or 1 normal cytology test and a negative HPV test result. The 2016 ACOG guidelines support this approach and state that it is reasonable to screen women immune-compromised for non-HIV reasons similarly starting at age 21 years. They recommend that women exposed to diethylstilbestrol in utero be screened annually, with no rationale provided.

CURRENT SCREENING STRATEGIES: LOW-RISK WOMEN

Women who have had surgical removal of the cervix have no risk of cervical cancer. Thus, current guidelines discourage screening among women after hysterectomy with no prior history of high-grade CIN or cancer. The USPSTF gives this a grade D recommendation (harms outweigh benefits). In women with high-grade CIN, ACOG recommends continued routine screening with cytology every 3 years for 20 years after the initial posttreatment surveillance period. This recommendation is more conservative than their 2003 recommendation suggesting screening cessation after 3 normal annual vaginal cytology tests.

Although it is anticipated that HPV vaccination will reduce the incidence of CIN and cancers, the lack of evidence of effectiveness at the population level has led guideline groups to recommend no change in the screening approach to vaccinated women. A recent decision analysis suggests that delaying screening initiation among vaccinated women and continuing with screening less often than every 3 years would be a cost-effective approach.[11]

CONTROVERSIES

Cancer screening guidelines are designed to maximize benefits and minimize harms, all at a reasonable cost. Frequent screening, earlier ages to begin, later ages to end, and more sensitive tests all contribute to screening effectiveness but, if untethered, also exacerbate screening harms and contribute to low-value care. Although current guidelines largely align, there is no consensus as to whether one screening approach should be preferred to another. ACS/ASCCP/ASCP recommend that cytology plus hrHPV testing (cotesting) should be preferred to cytology alone, although the guidelines' authors acknowledge that the evidence supporting the preferred designation is weak. ACOG agrees, justifying cotesting rather than cytology alone by citing evidence that hrHPV testing improves detection of adenocarcinoma. More simply, the USPSTF recommends this strategy be applied to women who would prefer screening less often that every 3 years.

The lack of head-to-head comparisons of cotesting with cytology alone with follow-up algorithms similar to those used in the United States has led to uncertainty with regard to expected outcomes. One Italian trial of 11,810 women aged 25 to 34 years randomized to conventional cytology or liquid-based cytology plus hrHPV testing yielded important results.[23] After 1 screening round, 17.3% of cotested women had either an abnormal cytology result or a positive hrHPV result compared with only 4.0% of women with cytology alone. However, despite such a large increase in positive testing, cotesting led to no additional cases of CIN3 identified but found substantially more cases of CIN1 and CIN2, lesions that are known to regress. Clearly age is an important factor in screening. Although the precise age before which hrHPV testing leads to more harms than benefits is unknown, all current guidelines discourage adding HPV testing to cytology in women less than age 30 years.

In 2014, the US Food and Drug Administration (FDA) approved a stand-alone hrHPV test for primary screening in women aged 25 years and older; this test detects the presence of 1 or more of 14 high-risk HPV types. In response to concerns about excessive colposcopy rates among those testing positive, the approved algorithm triages to colposcopy only those with evidence of HPV types 16 and 18 as well as those with evidence of the 12 other high-risk types who have abnormal cytology. After adjusting for verification bias, the study on which the guideline is based found that colposcopy of everyone with positive hrHPV tests had a sensitivity of 61% for CIN2+; triage with testing for HPV types 16 and 18 reduced the proportion of women undergoing colposcopy but at the expense of sensitivity (45%).[24] It is recommended that women with abnormal tests who do not proceed to colposcopy (eg, those with evidence of the 12 other high-risk types who have concurrent normal cytology) have follow-up in 1 year.[25]

The FDA-approved start age of 25 year for stand-alone hrHPV testing is controversial because it contradicts current recommendations by the USPSTF that discourage HPV testing in women less than age 30 years, reflecting the concern that the high prevalence of HPV infection in this age group will lead to oversurveillance and overtreatment. In the study cited earlier, 21% of women aged 25 to 29 years had positive HPV tests and were referred to colposcopy or placed in surveillance compared with about 7% screened with cytology alone.[24]

EMERGING NOVEL SCREENING STRATEGIES

Other novel strategies incorporate hrHPV testing as a first-line stand-alone test. An ongoing trial in Canada (the FOCAL trial) is now randomizing women into 2 arms: (1) hrHPV testing with reflex cytology for those testing positive (women with abnormal cytology get colposcopy), and (2) cytology with reflex hrHPV testing for those ASC-US (women with ASC-US cytology and positive hrHPV testing or LSIL cytology or worse get colposcopy). After a single round, the primary hrHPV screening arm detected more cases of CIN2+ (16.5 out of 1000 vs 10.1 out of 1000) and CIN3+ (7.5 out of 1000 vs 4.6 out of 1000), but required more women to have colposcopy compared with the control arm (58.9 out of 1000 vs 30.9 out of 1000).[26] Full trial results will provide important evidence on the reach, effectiveness, and cost-effectiveness of this strategy.

In addition to novel screening strategies, innovative screening techniques for hrHPV and cytology screening may be more acceptable to women, potentially broadening the reach among underscreened women. Specifically, self-collection of hrHPV removes the need for a speculum examination, a clinician, and possibly even a clinic visit. Self-collected hrHPV specimens have similar sensitivity and specificity for high-grade CIN to clinician-collected specimens.[27,28] Although most of the work in self-collection has been done in low-resource settings, multiple studies have shown self-collection to be highly acceptable to women in North America.[24,29–31] However, fewer studies have shown a relationship between self-collected HPV and increased screening rates or follow-up referral visits among underscreened women.[24] Studies of self-collection of cytology specimens have been limited to small pilots, likely because of the theoretic difficulty in obtaining endocervical cells using a vaginal swab and the increasing use of self-collection for HPV testing.

HIGH-VALUE SCREENING

Clinical guidelines strive to balance benefits and harms in an attempt to make screening high value, at least from the patient's perspective. Clinician surveys monitoring adherence to cervical cancer screening guidelines have been discouraging. In the past, clinicians have had low guidelines adherence,[32–34] including beginning screening too early[35]; repeating screening more often than indicated[35–38]; and not ending screening in low-risk women, either at age 65 years[32,39,40] or after hysterectomy for benign disease.[41,42] Recent studies show a more optimistic picture, suggesting that the age of screening initiation is increasing,[43] and screening visits for women aged 65 years and older are decreasing.[40] These changes could be caused by improved adherence to guidelines, patient acceptance of less screening, or changes in reimbursement for services that are not endorsed by guidelines.

Some aspects of cervical cancer screening have been the subject of the Healthcare Effectiveness Data and Information Set (HEDIS) of the National Committee for Quality Assurance. In 2014, a new performance measure entitled "Non-recommended cervical cancer screening in adolescent females" was proposed to capture unnecessary cervical cancer screening. Adding overscreening as a measure of poor-quality care by clinicians may bolster adherence to current guidelines.

Other definitions of high-value care consider costs more specifically. One major driver of overall costs is screening periodicity. When cervical cancer screening is conducted annually with either cytology alone or cytology in combination with HPV testing, the cost-effectiveness has been shown to exceed $500,000 per quality-adjusted life year (QALY) gained.[44,45] Biennial screening has been associated with incremental cost-effectiveness ratios of $150,000 to $200,000 per QALY gained,[44,46,47] in part because of the finding that most lesions detected at the frequent screening intervals are those that would regress if left undiscovered and untreated. In contrast, screening conducted every 3 to 5 years has been shown to be associated with less than $100,000 per QALY gained.[46,48] However, all QALY analyses to date have been limited by a lack of a comprehensive set of utilities capturing women's preferences for health states that follow from various strategies.[49]

EVIDENCE GAPS

It is useful to consider the 6 domains of health care quality put forth by the Institute of Medicine in 2001 when considering the way forward in cervical cancer screening. Clinicians strive to make care safe, effective, patient centered, timely, efficient, and equitable. As new strategies emerge, it will be useful to hold them to these standards to ensure that they are not just newer but also better. Patient-centeredness is key, and better understanding the patient's experience as she proceeds through the screening process will be valuable. Finding ways to make screening acceptable to hard-to-reach groups will realize the greatest impact of screening on cervical cancer incidence. Appropriate HPV vaccination holds great promise for additional protection, especially among sociodemographic groups that may be at risk of being unengaged in future screening settings.

SUMMARY

Cervical cancer screening in the United States has accompanied profound decreases in cancer incidence and mortality over the last half century. Maintaining gains in cervical cancer prevention requires a continued vigilant approach. Current screening guidelines issued by major groups are largely consistent and strive to find a reasonable balance between benefits and harms by recommending less than annual screening in most women. Attention to minimizing screening harms is an important aspect of all screening and preventive approaches.

As new screening strategies emerge and are adopted, comparative effectiveness analyses will be needed to outline the patient-centered and economic implications of choosing one rather than another. These analyses will be useful for highlighting high-value screening options to clinicians, health systems, and patients.[49] Above all, providing women with affordable, easily accessible screening, follow-up of abnormal tests, and timely treatment will result in the greatest impact of screening on cervical cancer incidence and mortality.

REFERENCES

1. Surveillance, Epidemiology, and End Results (SEER) Program of the National Cancer Institute. Available at: http://seer.cancer.gov/statfacts/html/cervix.html. Accessed November 26, 2016.
2. Centers for Disease Control and Prevention. Genital HPV infection fact sheet. Available at: http://www.cdc.gov/std/hpv/stdfact-hpv.htm. Accessed November 27, 2016.
3. Sawaya GF, Smith-McCune K. Cervical cancer screening. Obstet Gynecol 2016; 127(3):459–67.
4. Kyrgiou M, Koliopoulos G, Martin-Hirsch P, et al. Obstetric outcomes after conservative treatment for intraepithelial or early invasive cervical lesions: systematic review and meta-analysis. Lancet 2006;367(9509):489–98.
5. Kyrgiou M, Athanasiou A, Paraskevaidi M, et al. Adverse obstetric outcomes after local treatment for cervical preinvasive and early invasive disease according to cone depth: systematic review and meta-analysis. BMJ 2016;354:i3633.
6. Practice bulletin no. 157: cervical cancer screening and prevention. Obstet Gynecol 2016;127(1):e1–20.
7. Petrosky E, Bocchini JA Jr, Hariri S, et al. Use of 9-valent human papillomavirus (HPV) vaccine: updated HPV vaccination recommendations of the advisory committee on immunization practices. MMWR Morb Mortal Wkly Rep 2015;64(11):300–4.
8. Lu B, Kumar A, Castellsague X, et al. Efficacy and safety of prophylactic vaccines against cervical HPV infection and diseases among women: a systematic review & meta-analysis. BMC Infect Dis 2011;11:13.
9. Kjaer SK, Sigurdsson K, Iversen OE, et al. A pooled analysis of continued prophylactic efficacy of quadrivalent human papillomavirus (types 6/11/16/18) vaccine against high-grade cervical and external genital lesions. Cancer Prev Res (Phila) 2009;2(10):868–78.
10. Herrero R. Human papillomavirus (HPV) vaccines: limited cross-protection against additional HPV types. J Infect Dis 2009;199(7):919–22.
11. Kim JJ, Burger EA, Sy S, et al. Optimal cervical cancer screening in women vaccinated against human papillomavirus. J Natl Cancer Inst 2017;109(2):1–9.
12. Benard VB, Thomas CC, King J, et al. Vital signs: cervical cancer incidence, mortality, and screening - United States, 2007-2012. MMWR Morb Mortal Wkly Rep 2014;63(44):1004–9.

13. NIH consensus statement online 1996 April 1-3, 43(1): 1–38. Available at: https://consensus.nih.gov/1996/1996CervicalCancer102html.htm. Accessed on December 20, 2016.

14. Sawaya GF, Kulasingam S, Denberg TD, et al. Cervical cancer screening in average-risk women: best practice advice from the Clinical Guidelines Committee of the American College of Physicians. Ann Intern Med 2015;162(12):851–9.

15. Stoler MH, Schiffman M, Atypical Squamous Cells of Undetermined Significance-Low-grade Squamous Intraepithelial Lesion Triage Study Group. Interobserver reproducibility of cervical cytologic and histologic interpretations: realistic estimates from the ASCUS-LSIL Triage Study. JAMA 2001;285(11):1500–5.

16. Vesco KK, Whitlock EP, Eder M, et al. Screening for cervical cancer: a systematic evidence review for the U.S. Preventive Services Task Force. Rockville (MD); Available at: https://www.ncbi.nlm.nih.gov/pubmed/22132428. Accessed May, 2011.

17. Arbyn M, Roelens J, Simoens C, et al. Human papillomavirus testing versus repeat cytology for triage of minor cytological cervical lesions. Cochrane Database Syst Rev 2013;(3):CD008054.

18. Committee on Practice Bulletins—Gynecology. ACOG practice bulletin number 131: Screening for cervical cancer. Obstet Gynecol 2012;120(5):1222–38.

19. Moyer VA. Screening for cervical cancer: U.S. Preventive Services Task Force recommendation statement. Ann Intern Med 2012;156(12):880–91. W312.

20. Saslow D, Solomon D, Lawson HW, et al. American Cancer Society, American Society for Colposcopy and Cervical Pathology, and American Society for Clinical Pathology screening guidelines for the prevention and early detection of cervical cancer. CA Cancer J Clin 2012;62(3):147–72.

21. Kulasingam SL, Havrilesky L, Ghebre R, et al. Screening for cervical cancer: a decision analysis for the U.S. Preventive Services Task Force. AHRQ publication no. 11-05157-EF-1. Rockville (MD): Agency for Healthcare Research and Quality; 2011.

22. Panel on Opportunistic Infections in HIV-Infected Adults and Adolescents. Guidelines for the prevention and treatment of opportunistic infections in HIV-infected adults and adolescents: recommendations from the Centers for Disease Control and Prevention, the National Institutes of Health, and the HIV Medicine Association of the Infectious Diseases Society of America. Available at: http://aidsinfo.nih.gov/contentfiles/lvguidelines/adult_oi.pdf. Accessed November 29, 2016.

23. Ronco G, Giorgi-Rossi P, Carozzi F, et al. Human papillomavirus testing and liquid-based cytology in primary screening of women younger than 35 years: results at recruitment for a randomised controlled trial. Lancet Oncol 2006;7(7): 547–55.

24. Duke P, Godwin M, Ratnam S, et al. Effect of vaginal self-sampling on cervical cancer screening rates: a community-based study in Newfoundland. BMC Womens Health 2015;15:47.

25. Huh WK, Ault KA, Chelmow D, et al. Use of primary high-risk human papillomavirus testing for cervical cancer screening: interim clinical guidance. J Low Genit Tract Dis 2015;19:91–6.

26. Ogilvie GS, Krajden M, van Niekerk D, et al. HPV for cervical cancer screening (HPV FOCAL): complete round 1 results of a randomized trial comparing HPV-based primary screening to liquid-based cytology for cervical cancer. Int J Cancer 2017;140(2):440–8.

27. Chen Q, Du H, Zhang R, et al. Evaluation of novel assays for the detection of human papilloma virus in self-collected samples for cervical cancer screening. Genet Mol Res 2016;15(2).

28. Ogilvie GS, Patrick DM, Schulzer M, et al. Diagnostic accuracy of self collected vaginal specimens for human papillomavirus compared to clinician collected human papillomavirus specimens: a meta-analysis. Sex Transm Infect 2005;81(3): 207–12.

29. Crosby RA, Hagensee ME, Vanderpool R, et al. Community-based screening for cervical cancer: a feasibility study of rural Appalachian women. Sex Transm Dis 2015;42(11):607–11.

30. Scarinci IC, Litton AG, Garces-Palacio IC, et al. Acceptability and usability of self-collected sampling for HPV testing among African-American women living in the Mississippi Delta. Womens Health Issues 2013;23(2):e123–30.

31. De Alba I, Anton-Culver H, Hubbell FA, et al. Self-sampling for human papillomavirus in a community setting: feasibility in Hispanic women. Cancer Epidemiol Biomarkers Prev 2008;17(8):2163–8.

32. Saint M, Gildengorin G, Sawaya GF. Current cervical neoplasia screening practices of obstetrician/gynecologists in the US. Am J Obstet Gynecol 2005; 192(2):414–21.

33. Corbelli J, Borrero S, Bonnema R, et al. Differences among primary care physicians' adherence to 2009 ACOG guidelines for cervical cancer screening. J Womens Health (Larchmt) 2013;23:397–403.

34. Perkins RB, Jorgensen JR, McCoy ME, et al. Adherence to conservative management recommendations for abnormal Pap test results in adolescents. Obstet Gynecol 2012;119(6):1157–63.

35. Roland KB, Soman A, Benard VB, et al. Human papillomavirus and Papanicolaou tests screening interval recommendations in the United States. Am J Obstet Gynecol 2011;205(5)(447):e441–8.

36. Berkowitz Z, Saraiya M, Sawaya GF. Cervical cancer screening intervals, 2006 to 2009: moving beyond annual testing. JAMA Int Med 2013;173(10):922–4.

37. Meissner HI, Tiro JA, Yabroff KR, et al. Too much of a good thing? Physician practices and patient willingness for less frequent pap test screening intervals. Med Care 2010;48(3):249–59.

38. Saraiya M, Berkowitz Z, Yabroff KR, et al. Cervical cancer screening with both human papillomavirus and Papanicolaou testing vs Papanicolaou testing alone: what screening intervals are physicians recommending? Arch Intern Med 2010; 170(11):977–85.

39. Bellizzi KM, Breslau ES, Burness A, et al. Prevalence of cancer screening in older, racially diverse adults: still screening after all these years. Arch Intern Med 2011; 171(22):2031–7.

40. Kale MS, Bishop TF, Federman AD, et al. Trends in the overuse of ambulatory health care services in the United States. JAMA Int Med 2013;173(2):142–8.

41. Cervical cancer screening among women by hysterectomy status and among women aged ≥65 years - United States, 2000-2010. MMWR Morb Mortal Wkly Rep 2013;61(51–52):1043–7.

42. Sirovich BE, Welch HG. Cervical cancer screening among women without a cervix. JAMA 2004;291(24):2990–3.

43. Henderson JT, Saraiya M, Martinez G, et al. Changes to cervical cancer prevention guidelines: effects on screening among U.S. women ages 15-29. Prev Med 2013;56(1):25–9.

44. Goldie SJ, Kim JJ, Wright TC. Cost-effectiveness of human papillomavirus DNA testing for cervical cancer screening in women aged 30 years or more. Obstet Gynecol 2004;103(4):619–31.
45. Kim JJ, Wright TC, Goldie SJ. Cost-effectiveness of alternative triage strategies for atypical squamous cells of undetermined significance. JAMA 2002;287(18): 2382–90.
46. Goldhaber-Fiebert JD, Stout NK, Salomon JA, et al. Cost-effectiveness of cervical cancer screening with human papillomavirus DNA testing and HPV-16,18 vaccination. J Natl Cancer Inst 2008;100(5):308–20.
47. Mandelblatt JS, Lawrence WF, Womack SM, et al. Benefits and costs of using HPV testing to screen for cervical cancer. JAMA 2002;287(18):2372–81.
48. Kim JJ, Sharma M, Ortendahl J. Optimal interval for routine cytologic screening in the United States. JAMA Int Med 2013;173(3):241–2.
49. Sawaya GF, Kuppermann M. Identifying a "range of reasonable options" for cervical cancer screening. Obstet Gynecol 2015;125(2):308–10.

Colorectal Cancer Screening in Average Risk Patients

Alison T. Brenner, PhD, MPH[a],*, Michael Dougherty, MD[b],
Daniel S. Reuland, MD, MPH[c]

KEYWORDS

- Colorectal cancer screening • Prevention • Implementation

KEY POINTS

- Colorectal cancer (CRC) is the third most common cause of cancer death in the United States, occurring primarily in individuals over the age of 50.
- Current evidence suggests that any of several recommended screening strategies can effectively reduce CRC mortality; commonly used approaches are primary endoscopic visualization procedures (colonoscopy and flexible sigmoidoscopy), and fecal tests for occult blood.
- Screening strategies vary with respect to their associated benefits, harms, costs, and patient experience. Offering patients stool-based screening is important for increasing screening uptake.
- Rather than a single test, CRC screening should be viewed as a cascade of events that must occur with fidelity in order for screening to be effective.
- A high-quality screening program requires substantial infrastructure to systematically identify the population at risk, provide education and decision support, and promote test ordering and completion; for fecal tests, systematic support facilitates adherence to regular testing as well as follow-up of abnormal tests.

INTRODUCTION

Colorectal cancer (CRC) is the third leading cause of cancer mortality among both men and women in the United States.[1] In 2016, 134,490 new cases of and 49,190 deaths from CRC are expected, with about 90% occurring in adults over the age of 50.[2] CRC

Disclosure Statement: Dr Dougherty was supported, in part, by a grant from the NIH (T32 DK007634).

[a] Cecil G Sheps Center for Health Services Research, University of North Carolina, 725 Martin Luther King Jr Boulevard, CB# 7590, Chapel Hill, NC 27599-7590, USA; [b] Division of Gastroenterology and Hepatology, Department of Medicine, University of North Carolina, 4182 Bioinformatics Building, 130 Mason Farm Road, Chapel Hill, NC 27599-6134, USA; [c] Division of General Internal Medicine, Department of Medicine, University of North Carolina, 725 Martin Luther King Jr Boulevard, CB# 7590, Chapel Hill, NC 27599-7590, USA
* Corresponding author.
E-mail address: alison.brenner@unc.edu

typically has a long, detectable latent period, making it a good candidate for screening. Screening for CRC has been shown to be both effective at reducing mortality and cost-effective from a societal perspective.[3] However, CRC screening is underutilized, particularly among vulnerable populations, including racial/ethnic minorities and groups with low socioeconomic status.[4] Multiple guidelines recommend that adults aged 50 to 75 complete regular screening.[1,5,6] Principal tests currently in use in the United States include colonoscopy and fecal occult blood testing (guaiac-based [gFOBT] and immunochemical [FIT]).[7]

In this article, the authors review risk factors for CRC, current screening recommendations from North American guideline organizations, and some of the tradeoffs associated with different screening strategies. Finally, the article describes key elements of a high-quality clinical screening program and reviews interventions shown to be successful at improving CRC screening.

BIOLOGICAL RATIONALE FOR SCREENING

CRC can develop through several molecular pathways, described in detail in other focused reviews.[8–10] A stepwise accumulation of mutations in tumor suppressor and oncogenes leads to chromosomal instability in colorectal epithelial cells and the formation of precursor adenomatous polyps, which progress through higher grades of dysplasia to eventual carcinoma. This sequence typically takes place over 10 years or longer, forming the basis for screening recommendations for colonoscopic examination with removal of all visible adenomas every 10 years.[11] Stool-based tests rely on the propensity of adenomas to bleed with more advanced size and neoplasia, allowing detection of most polyps and/or cancers while they are still easily treatable.[12,13] Although this paradigm has proven useful for reducing CRC mortality,[12] alternate carcinogenesis pathways, such as microsatellite instability and the serrated polyp pathway, can deviate from this sequence, often manifesting as right-sided, difficult-to-visualize lesions that may bleed less in earlier stages and progress through the polyp-to-carcinoma sequence in under 10 years.[8,10,14]

RISK FACTORS

Modifiable risk factors for CRC include heavy smoking, heavy alcohol intake, red and processed meat consumption, physical inactivity, and obesity.[15] Dietary fiber, calcium, folate, and fish oil are associated with lower CRC risk, although interventions targeting these associations have been disappointing.[16] Nonmodifiable risk factors include familial risk, male sex, older age, and race/ethnicity. Socioeconomic status and other barriers to health care access likely mediate the most increased incidence in minorities,[17] although African Americans may also possess independent elevated risk.[18] Ashkenazi Jewish populations are also at higher risk, due to high prevalence of adenomatous polyposis coli gene mutations.[19] The effect size of nonfamilial, nonsyndromic risk is generally too small to alter guideline recommendations for screening, although the American College of Gastroentrology (ACG) recommends screening African Americans from age 45.[20]

Familial and Genetic Risk

The genetic basis for most familial risk is not well characterized, and although only elevating risk 2- to 4-fold, contributes to 20% to 25% of incident CRC in the general population.[21] Having a first- or second-degree relative with CRC or even a history of adenomatous polyps increases one's risk and often affects screening recommendations. Risk increases with number of family members, closer relation, and younger age at diagnosis as well as presence of cancer versus adenoma alone.[21] The extreme of familial risk is the set of well-defined, monogenetic hereditary cancer syndromes, increasing lifetime risk from 10% (Cowden syndrome) to nearly 100% (classic familial adenomatous polyposis).[22]

A hereditary cancer syndrome should be suspected based on personal or family history of multiple malignancies and/or suggestive endoscopic findings. Evidence is lacking on the optimal timing of obtaining a complete family cancer history for the average medical patient, but experts recommend a minimum initial query at 20 years of age, so that patients with cancer syndromes may have timely referral for genetic counseling, confirmatory testing, and the corresponding colonoscopic screening programs.[22,23] The history should include the types and ages of onset of any cancers in first- or second-degree relatives[22] and should be confirmed or updated periodically (some have suggested an interval of every 5–10 years).[24] Regarding nonsyndromic familial risk, a history of CRC in multiple first-degree relatives (FDRs), or any FDR younger than 60, warrants commencement of earlier screening. Experts recommend that these patients receive colonoscopy (rather than other screening methods) at an interval of every 5 years, starting at age 40 or 10 years before the age of the relative's diagnosis, whichever comes first.[20,25]

Other Medical Conditions

Several non-Mendelian medical conditions also appear to influence CRC risk, including type 2 diabetes,[26] prior cholecystectomy,[27] prior cytotoxic chemotherapy or abdominal radiation,[8,28] and prolonged immunosuppression,[29] although it is unclear if and how these should affect screening recommendations. Acromegaly and prior ureterosigmoidostomy[8] present progressively greater risks, but the medical condition that contributes the most increased risk at the population level is inflammatory bowel disease (IBD: Crohn disease, ulcerative colitis).[30] Patients with IBD should be screened with colonoscopy beginning 8 years after diagnosis, except for cases of ulcerative proctitis or proctosigmoiditis, which can be screened according to average-risk population guidelines.[30]

TESTS USED FOR SCREENING

In 2016, the USPSTF reviewed evidence regarding the benefits and harms of screening approaches, including colonoscopy, flexible sigmoidoscopy (FSIG), computed tomography colonography (CTC), gFOBT, FIT, and the multitargeted stool DNA test. The task force concluded with "high certainty" that CRC screening in average-risk adults aged 50 to 75 years was substantially beneficial. They found that multiple, effective screening strategies were available and that each was supported by different levels of evidence, with unique advantages and disadvantages.[11]

Benefits and Harms of Different Screening Approaches

To help formulate recommendations, the US Preventive Services Task Force (USPSTF) commissioned modeling studies to compare the benefits and harms of different screening strategies. Benefits of screening were measured using life years gained (LYG) and reduction in incidence and mortality from CRC. To assess harms, modelers used the lifetime number of colonoscopies required (colonoscopy burden) as a proxy for the morbidity and cost associated with each screening strategy.[3] The models suggested that the following screening strategies were the most "efficient" in terms of optimizing LYG per additional colonoscopy: annual FIT, annual FIT plus FSIG every 10 years, primary colonoscopy every 10 years, and CTC every 5 years.[3]

However, although CTC was found to be efficient by these measures, the task force noted a lack of evidence regarding other potentially important harms of CTC, particularly with respect to incidental extracolonic findings and radiation exposure.[3,11] In later discussion, the authors briefly summarize modeled projections of the key benefits (LYG and deaths averted) and harms (colonoscopy burden) accruing in 1000 individuals screened using 4 of the most common screening approaches: FIT, gFOBT, FIT + FSIG, and colonoscopy (**Table 1**).

Annual gFOBT and FIT are projected to provide similar benefits, but FIT, being as sensitive and more specific than gFOBT, would result in somewhat fewer lifetime colonoscopies. FIT also offers some advantages over gFOBT in terms of the process for test completion; some FIT assays require only one sample (instead of 3 with gFOBT), a feature that can improve adherence.[31] FSIG every 10 years paired with annual FIT achieves a slightly higher mortality benefit than gFOBT/FIT alone, but results in more lifetime colonoscopies, and thus more potential for colonoscopy-related complications. Colonoscopy every 10 years as a primary screening strategy achieves the largest morbidity and mortality benefit of the recommended screening strategies. However, it also requires substantial preparation and recovery time,[32] leads to the highest number of lifetime colonoscopies (more than 2-fold that of FIT), and, thus, the highest rate of complications following screening.

Cost of Testing

All USPSTF-recommended screening tests are covered at full cost under the Affordable Care Act.[33] However, cost to patients associated with different strategies will vary highly depending on insurance type and test results, because abnormal results lead to additional or more frequent testing.

SCREENING GUIDELINES

For average-risk adults, North American guideline organizations are largely concordant with the USPSTF on recommendations of multiple screening strategies (**Table 2**). Guidelines differ primarily on inclusion and relative strength of recommendation for colonoscopy, CTC, gFOBT, and stool DNA tests, as well as whether pairing FSIG with a program of stool-based testing provides a worthwhile advantage over FSIG alone.[11,20,25,34,35] All guidelines recommend colonoscopy for follow-up of any abnormal noncolonoscopy screening test. Patients with adenomatous polyps on endoscopy should be followed under a published surveillance protocol.[36] Patients with only 1 or 2 small (≤10 mm) tubular adenomas on initial colonoscopy are at low risk for CRC and require a surveillance interval of 5 to 10 years.[36]

The ACG endorses a colonoscopy-based strategy as part of an overall preference for cancer "prevention" tests over cancer "detection" tests, and an alternative to the "menu of options" approach of the USMSTF.[20] The Canadian guidelines round out the other end of the spectrum, emphasizing randomized controlled trial level evidence and availability in Canada in their endorsement of only fecal tests or FSIG, and recommending against CTC or primary colonoscopy.[35] Starting age for average-risk individuals is 50 years according to all guidelines.

Screening in Older Adults and Those with Limited Life Expectancy

Guidelines generally recommend against CRC screening adults over the age of 85.[11,20,34,35,37] For adults between the ages of 75 and 85 who have previously completed regular screening, life expectancy should be considered in screening cessation decisions. Patients with life-expectancy of less than 5 to 10 years are

Table 1
Test performance and other characteristics of commonly performed colorectal cancer screening tests, per 1000 people screened

	Sensitivity/ Specificity[a,b]	LYG[b]	CRC Cases Averted (%)[b]	CRC Deaths Averted (%)[b]	Lifetime Colonoscopies[b]	Complications[e]	Nature of Test
gFOBT (1 y)	62%–79% 87%–96%	232–261	33–54 (49%–75%)	20–23 (73%–82%)	2230–2287	11	No preparation, no recovery time, 3 stool samples, completed at home yearly
FIT (1 y)	10-μg cutoff: 79%–88% 91%–93% 20-μg cutoff: 73%–75% 91%–95%	231–260	31–52 (47%–72%)	20–23 (72%–81%)	1739–1899	10–11	No preparation, no recovery time, 1 stool sample, completed at home yearly
FIT-DNA (3 y)	92% 84%	215–250	29–49 (43%–68%)	19–22 (68%–78%)	1701–1827	9–10	No preparation, no recovery time, 1 stool sample, completed at home every 3 y
FSIG (10 y) FIT (1 y)	FSIG 60%–70% as sensitive COLO[c]	246–270	38–57 (76%–85%)	22–24 (77%–85%)	2248–2490	11–12	FSIG: ½ day prep time, 1 h recovery time, completed every 10 y in a medical facility
COLO (10 y)	Reference	248–275	42–63 (62%–88%)	22–24 (79%–90%)	4007–4101	14–15	24 h prep time, 1 d recovery time, completed every 10 y in a medical facility
CTC (5 y)	67%–94% 85%–98%[d]	226–265	34–56 (51%–78%)	20–24 (72%–85%)	1654–1927	10–11	24 h prep time, 1 h recovery time, completed every 5 y in a medical facility

[a] Per 1 time use of test.
[b] Knudsen, 2016; Zauber 2015; USPSTF 2016.
[c] Operator dependent, no evidence comparing FSIG directly to COLO.
[d] Sensitivity and specificity for detecting adenomas ≥10 mm.
[e] Complications include gastrointestinal events (eg, bleeding, perforation) and cardiopulmonary events (eg, myocardial infarction, angina, cardiac/respiratory arrest).

Table 2
Comparison of colorectal cancer screening recommendations of North American guidelines committees

	USPSTF	ACG	MSTF/ACS/ACR	ACP	CPSTF
Recommendations	• Colonoscopy every 10 y • CTC every 5 y[a] • FSIG every 10 y plus FIT every year • gFOBT[b] or FIT	Preferred: • Colonoscopy every 10 y First alternatives: • CTC every 5 y • FS every 5–10 y • FIT every year Acceptable when all other options declined or unavailable: • gFOBT[b] annually or stool DNA every 3 y	• Colonoscopy every 10 y • CTC every 5 y • FSIG every 5 y • DCBE every 5 y • gFOBT,[b] FIT every year • Stool DNA at uncertain intervals, but more frequent than every 5 y[c]	• Colonoscopy every 10 y • FSIG every 5 y • FSIG every 5 y plus FIT or gFOBT[b] every 3 y • gFOBT[b] or FIT every year	• FSIG every 10 y • gFOBT[b] or FIT every 2 y
Starting age, average risk	50	50, except 45 in African Americans	50	50	50–60[d]
Stopping age[e]	75–85, depending on individual risk, life-expectancy, and values	Not discussed	Not discussed	75–85, depending on individual risk, life-expectancy, and values	75

Abbreviations: ACR, American College of Radiology; ACS, American Cancer Society; DCBE, double contrast barium enema; FSIG, flexible sigmoidoscopy; MSTF, Multi-Society Task Force.

[a] Only equivalent to other strategies if the burden of screening metric is lifetime colonoscopies, not lifetime cathartic bowel preparations. Does not account for possible risks of frequent, low-dose radiation, or incidental extra-colonic findings.
[b] Should always be "high-sensitivity" (eg, Hemoccult Sensa) guaiac-based test if used.
[c] Combined FIT-DNA test not available at time of publication.
[d] Canadian guidelines weight recommendation strength by age, with ages 50 to 59 receiving a "weak" recommendation for screening, and ages 60 to 74 a "strong" recommendation.
[e] Assuming personal history of appropriate screening without diagnosis of a high-risk condition.

unlikely to benefit from additional CRC screening, as the mortality benefit does not begin to accrue for at least 5 years after initiation.[38] Furthermore, the risk of severe complications, such as a severe gastrointestinal bleeding after polypectomy, is increased in older populations. When the balance of benefits and harms is unclear, decisions about stopping screening should be made through a shared decision-making process, incorporating life expectancy, comorbidity, and patient preference.

IMPLEMENTATION CONSIDERATIONS
Features of a High-Quality Screening Program

CRC screening should be viewed as a program of coordinated steps, rather than a single screening test. These steps must occur reliably in order for screening to reduce CRC mortality. A high-quality CRC screening program should deliver appropriate screening to a substantial proportion of patients by using both visit-based and non-visit-based protocols that *systematically* ensure the following steps occur:

1. Identification of patients due for either initial or repeat screening, including identifying those in the higher CRC risk tiers
2. Patient education about screening, including decision support if more than one screening option is available to patients
3. Test ordering
4. Tracking of ordered screening tests and providing sufficient patient support to ensure test completion
5. Follow-up of abnormal screening findings and adherence to repeat screening

Which test or tests to offer

As recognized by recent USPSTF guidelines, there is no direct evidence that one screening approach is clearly superior to others, particularly when colonoscopy burden, cost, availability, patient preferences, and adherence are considered.[11] In fact, although colonoscopy has been the dominant primary screening strategy in the United States in recent years and is widely viewed as the most effective *single* CRC screening test, emerging evidence suggests that patients' screening preferences and adherence are critical factors determining the impact a screening *program* will have on CRC mortality. For example, recent interim analysis of a European trial directly comparing colonoscopy and FIT-based strategies found that individuals initially invited for FIT-based strategy were more likely to participate in screening than were those initially invited for colonoscopy screening, resulting in an equal number of early-stage CRCs detected in each study arm.[39] Furthermore, accumulating evidence from studies in North America suggests that offering stool testing with gFOBT or FIT is a key to increasing screening rates. For example, Inadomi and colleagues[40] found that offering colonoscopy alone yielded a lower screening completion rate (38%) compared with offering gFOBT/FIT alone (67%) or a choice of either test (69%), in vulnerable patients.

Decision aids

One way to systematically and explicitly offer a choice of screening tests is by using a patient decision aid. Trials of decision aids show they increase screening-related knowledge, intent, and test ordering.[41] Decision aids have also been shown to increase screening completion, although the effect is typically modest (about 8% points vs usual care).[42]

Patient navigation

In this context, the term "patient navigation" can refer broadly to interventions delivered by nonphysicians to help patients overcome barriers to CRC screening. Patient navigators can be linked to clinical practices, health systems, community organizations, or payers. Accumulating evidence suggests that patient navigation is a promising intervention that is particularly helpful in increasing CRC screening in vulnerable populations.[43–47]

Other strategies

Other visit-based and non-visit-based strategies have been shown to be effective in improving screening rates within practices and integrated systems.[48] Visit-based strategies can include reminder systems to help care teams identify patients due for screening.[49,50] Practices should consider creating standing orders that permit nonphysician team members to offer and track the return of gFOBT/FIT kits without requiring physician orders for individual patients. Other strategies that have been shown to improve screening rates include offering screening during nurse-driven influenza vaccination clinics.[51] Non-visit-based outreach to patients due for screening, including mailed reminders with or without FIT kits, or mailing gFOBT cards timed to a scheduled clinic appointment, can increase screening.[52–55]

Combined interventions

Considering the steps involved in the CRC screening process and the heterogeneity of populations and health system delivery contexts in North America, it is doubtful that any single intervention type will lead to high rates of CRC screening adherence in a given practice, community, or region. Instead, complementary interventions designed to address barriers at different steps along the screening process are likely to yield larger impacts than single interventions.

Adherence to repeat guaiac-based fecal occult blood test/fecal immunochemical test testing and follow-up of abnormal results

To reduce CRC mortality, gFOBT or FIT testing should be done annually, or at least biennially. Without systems to support repeat testing, adherence to these stool-based programs is likely to be suboptimal. For example, a follow-up study of a successful CRC screening intervention trial found a substantial reduction in adherence to stool-based screening in the years after the active intervention was removed.[56] Conversely, other studies have shown that adherence to stool testing can be maintained at high-level interventions through use of interventions such as mailed reminders and telephone/text outreach.[57] Ensuring high rates of follow-up of abnormal stool screening tests for CRC is also critical for stool-based screening regimens to be effective. Patient navigation and programs of physician-directed reminder feedback plus academic detailing can increase diagnostic resolution of abnormal screening stool tests.[58,59]

The importance of team-based care

Regardless of which screening implementation strategies are chosen, competing demands currently experienced by primary care providers requires that nonphysicians be enlisted as part of a team-based, systematic approach to CRC screening.[60] Although CRC screening is widely understood to represent high-value care from a societal perspective, fee-for-service payment models have not traditionally reimbursed primary practices for staff time needed for systematic screening activities, such as visit planning, registry development and maintenance, outreach, and navigation. It is hoped that changes in payment models will provide primary care "medical homes" with the resources required to implement high-quality CRC screening programs.

Overuse of screening

Unfortunately, in addition to substantial underuse of CRC screening overall, there is also evidence of overuse of screening in patient populations unlikely to derive net benefit from screening due to advanced age or comorbidities.[61–65]

CRC screening programs should incorporate systems that take into account not only a patents' risk of CRC but also life expectancy, health status, and individual preferences.

PRIMARY PREVENTION

Although no primary prevention strategy is so effective as to obviate screening, the understanding of primary prevention strategies is evolving.

Aspirin

Aspirin appears to reduce the risk of CRC and adenomas after 5 to 10 years of use, although its use for this indication has been controversial because of the associated bleeding risks. Nevertheless, because aspirin also prevents cardiovascular disease (CVD) events, the USPSTF recommended in 2016 that low-dose aspirin be used for the primary prevention of CVD and CRC in adults aged 50 to 59 years who have a 10% or greater 10-year CVD risk, are not at increased risk for bleeding, have a life expectancy of at least 10 years, and are willing to take low-dose aspirin daily for at least 10 years (grade B recommendation).[66]

Lifestyle and Diet

Despite lack of robust trial evidence for the effect on CRC incidence of modifying life-style risk factors, the general health and cardiovascular benefits of avoiding smoking, heavy alcohol use, weight gain, and physical inactivity allow for strong recommendations for these behaviors. Likewise, experts recommend CRC risk reduction by replacing red meat, processed foods, and refined starches in the diet with poultry, fish, and plant sources as the primary source of protein; unsaturated fats as the primary source of fat; and unrefined grains, legumes, and fruits as the primary source of carbohydrates.[67]

SUMMARY

CRC contributes a major burden of cancer mortality in North America. Although there are multiple effective screening approaches that can reduce CRC mortality, screening remains underused. Implementation of systematic, population-based screening interventions that address multiple steps involved in the screening process is a key to improving CRC screening rates. In planning for implementation, decision makers should consider the overall impact of screening *programs* (rather than individual screening tests) as well as factors such as adherence, patient preferences, and available resources. Offering patients stool-based testing with gFOBT/FIT is likely to improve uptake compared with offering colonoscopy alone. However, programs that offer stool testing must include the population health infrastructure needed to promote adherence to repeat testing and follow-up of abnormal tests.

ACKNOWLEDGMENTS

The authors to thank Jim Evans, MD, PhD for suggestions regarding screening for genetic risk for CRC.

REFERENCES

1. American Cancer Society. Cancer Facts & Figures. American Cancer Society; 2016:12.
2. SEER. Cancer of the Colon and Rectum - SEER Stat Fact Sheets. 2016. Available at: https://seer.cancer.gov/statfacts/html/colorect.html. Accessed November 28, 2016.
3. Knudsen AB, Zauber AG, Rutter CM, et al. Estimation of benefits, burden, and harms of colorectal cancer screening strategies: modeling study for the US Preventive Services Task Force. JAMA 2016;315(23):2595–609.
4. White A, Thompson TD, White MC, et al. Cancer Screening Test Use - United States 2015. MMWR Morb Mortal Wkly Rep 2017;66(8):205.
5. Healthy People 2020. 2016. Available at: https://www.healthypeople.gov/. Accessed November 30, 2016.
6. National Colorectal Cancer Roundtable. Shared Goal: Reaching 80% Screened for Colorectal Cancer by 2018. 2015. Available at: http://nccrt.org/wp-content/uploads/80by2018Commitment.pdf. Accessed March 3, 2015.
7. Centers for Disease Control and Prevention (CDC). Vital signs: colorectal cancer screening test use - United States 2012. MMWR Morb Mortal Wkly Rep 2013; 62(44):881–8.
8. Cappell MS. Pathophysiology, clinical presentation, and management of colon cancer. Gastroenterol Clin North Am 2008;37(1):1–24.
9. Biswas S, Holyoake D, Maughan TS. Molecular taxonomy and tumourigenesis of colorectal cancer. Clin Oncol (R Coll Radiol) 2016;28(2):73–82.
10. Leggett B, Whitehall V. Role of the serrated pathway in colorectal cancer pathogenesis. Gastroenterology 2010;138(6):2088–100.
11. U.S. Preventive Services Task Force, Bibbins-Domingo K, Grossman DC, et al. Screening for colorectal cancer: US Preventive Services Task Force recommendation statement. JAMA 2016;315(23):2564–75.
12. Lin JS, Piper MA, Perdue LA, et al. Screening for colorectal cancer: updated evidence report and systematic review for the us preventive services task force. JAMA 2016;315(23):2576–94.
13. Robertson DJ, Lee JK, Boland CR, et al. Recommendations on fecal immuno-chemical testing to screen for colorectal neoplasia: a consensus statement by the US Multi-Society Task Force on colorectal cancer. Gastrointest Endosc 2016;85:2–21.e3.
14. Nishihara R, Wu K, Lochhead P, et al. Long-term colorectal-cancer incidence and mortality after lower endoscopy. N Engl J Med 2013;369(12):1095–105.
15. Huxley RR, Ansary-Moghaddam A, Clifton P, et al. The impact of dietary and lifestyle risk factors on risk of colorectal cancer: a quantitative overview of the epidemiological evidence. Int J Cancer 2009;125(1):171–80.
16. Cooper K, Squires H, Carroll C, et al. Chemoprevention of colorectal cancer: systematic review and economic evaluation. Health Technol Assess 2010;14(32):1–206.
17. Lansdorp-Vogelaar I, Kuntz KM, Knudsen AB, et al. Contribution of screening and survival differences to racial disparities in colorectal cancer rates. Cancer Epidemiol Biomarkers Prev 2012;21(5):728–36.
18. Williams R, White P, Nieto J, et al. Colorectal cancer in African Americans: an update: prepared by the Committee on Minority Affairs and Cultural Diversity, American College of Gastroenterology. Clin Translational Gastroenterol 2016;7(7):e185.
19. Locker GY, Lynch HT. Genetic factors and colorectal cancer in Ashkenazi Jews. Fam Cancer 2004;3(3–4):215–21.

20. Rex DK, Johnson DA, Anderson JC, et al. American College of Gastroenterology guidelines for colorectal cancer screening 2009 [corrected]. Am J Gastroenterol 2009;104(3):739–50.

21. Lowery JT, Ahnen DJ, Schroy PC 3rd, et al. Understanding the contribution of family history to colorectal cancer risk and its clinical implications: a state-of-the-science review. Cancer 2016;122(17):2633–45.

22. Syngal S, Brand RE, Church JM, et al. ACG clinical guideline: genetic testing and management of hereditary gastrointestinal cancer syndromes. Am J Gastroenterol 2015;110(2):223–62.

23. Winawer S, Fletcher R, Rex D, et al. Colorectal cancer screening and surveillance: clinical guidelines and rationale-update based on new evidence. Gastroenterology 2003;124(2):544–60.

24. Ziogas A, Horick NK, Kinney AY, et al. Clinically relevant changes in family history of cancer over time. JAMA 2011;306(2):172–8.

25. Levin B, Lieberman DA, McFarland B, et al. Screening and surveillance for the early detection of colorectal cancer and adenomatous polyps, 2008: a joint guideline from the American Cancer Society, the US Multi-Society Task Force on Colorectal Cancer, and the American College of Radiology. Gastroenterology 2008;134(5):1570–95.

26. Yuhara H, Steinmaus C, Cohen SE, et al. Is diabetes mellitus an independent risk factor for colon cancer and rectal cancer? Am J Gastroenterol 2011;106(11): 1911–21 [quiz: 1922].

27. Lagergren J, Ye W, Ekbom A. Intestinal cancer after cholecystectomy: is bile involved in carcinogenesis? Gastroenterology 2001;121(3):542–7.

28. Henderson TO, Oeffinger KC, Whitton J, et al. Secondary gastrointestinal cancer in childhood cancer survivors: a cohort study. Ann Intern Med 2012;156(11): 757–66, w-260.

29. Johnson EE, Leverson GE, Pirsch JD, et al. A 30-year analysis of colorectal adenocarcinoma in transplant recipients and proposal for altered screening. J Gastrointest Surg 2007;11(3):272–9.

30. Farraye FA, Odze RD, Eaden J, et al. AGA technical review on the diagnosis and management of colorectal neoplasia in inflammatory bowel disease. Gastroenterology 2010;138(2):746–74, 774.e1–4; [quiz: e712–743].

31. Vart G, Banzi R, Minozzi S. Comparing participation rates between immunochemical and guaiac faecal occult blood tests: a systematic review and meta-analysis. Prev Med 2012;55(2):87–92.

32. Jonas DE, Russell LB, Sandler RS, et al. Patient time requirements for screening colonoscopy. Am J Gastroenterol 2007;102(11):2401–10.

33. Department of Health and Human Services. Preventive Services Covered Under the Affordable Care Act. Health Care Facts & Features 2010. Available at: https://www.hhs.gov/healthcare/facts-and-features/fact-sheets/preventive-services-covered-under-aca/. Accessed January 16, 2017.

34. Wilt TJ, Harris RP, Qaseem A, High value care task force of the American College of Physicians. Screening for cancer: advice for high-value care from the American College of Physicians. Ann Intern Med 2015;162(10):718–25.

35. Canadian Task Force on Preventive Health Care, Bacchus CM, Dunfield L, et al. Recommendations on screening for colorectal cancer in primary care. CMAJ 2016;188(5):340–8.

36. Lieberman DA, Rex DK, Winawer SJ, et al. Guidelines for colonoscopy surveillance after screening and polypectomy: a consensus update by the US Multi-Society Task Force on Colorectal Cancer. Gastroenterology 2012;143(3):844–57.

37. Ahlquist DA, Sargent DJ, Loprinzi CL, et al. Stool DNA and occult blood testing for screen detection of colorectal neoplasia. Ann Intern Med 2008;149(7):441–51.

38. Lansdorp-Vogelaar I, Gulati R, Mariotto AB, et al. Personalizing age of cancer screening cessation based on comorbid conditions: model estimates of harms and benefits. Ann Intern Med 2014;161(2):104–12.

39. Quintero E, Castells A, Bujanda L, et al. Colonoscopy versus fecal immunochemical testing in colorectal-cancer screening. N Engl J Med 2012;366(8):697–706.

40. Inadomi JM, Vijan S, Janz NK, et al. Adherence to colorectal cancer screening: a randomized clinical trial of competing strategies. Arch Intern Med 2012;172(7): 575–82.

41. Brenner AT, Hoffman R, McWilliams A, et al. Colorectal cancer screening in vulnerable patients: promoting informed and shared decisions. Am J Prev Med 2016;51:454–62.

42. Volk RJ, Linder SK, Lopez-Olivo MA, et al. Patient decision aids for colorectal cancer screening: a systematic review and meta-analysis. Am J Prev Med 2016;51:779–91.

43. Jandorf L, Braschi C, Ernstoff E, et al. Culturally targeted patient navigation for increasing African Americans' adherence to screening colonoscopy: a randomized clinical trial. Cancer Epidemiol Biomarkers Prev 2013;22(9):1577–87.

44. Percac-Lima S, Ashburner JM, Zai AH, et al. Patient navigation for comprehensive cancer screening in high-risk patients using a population-based health information technology system: a randomized clinical trial. JAMA Intern Med 2016; 176:930–7.

45. Percac-Lima S, Grant RW, Green AR, et al. A culturally tailored navigator program for colorectal cancer screening in a community health center: a randomized, controlled trial. J Gen Intern Med 2009;24(2):211–7.

46. Lasser KE, Murillo J, Lisboa S, et al. Colorectal cancer screening among ethnically diverse, low-income patients: a randomized controlled trial. Arch Intern Med 2011;171(10):906–12.

47. Lasser KE, Murillo J, Medlin E, et al. A multilevel intervention to promote colorectal cancer screening among community health center patients: results of a pilot study. BMC Fam Pract 2009;10:37.

48. Holden D, Jonas DE, Porterfield DSDS, et al. Systematic review: enhancing use and quality of colorectal cancer screening. Ann Intern Med 2010;152(10):668–76.

49. Sequist TD, Zaslavsky AM, Marshall R, et al. Patient and physician reminders to promote colorectal cancer screening: a randomized controlled trial. Arch Intern Med 2009;169(4):364–71.

50. Sabatino SA, Lawrence B, Elder R, et al. Effectiveness of interventions to increase screening for breast, cervical, and colorectal cancers: nine updated systematic reviews for the guide to community preventive services. Am J Prev Med 2012; 43(1):97–118.

51. Potter MB, Ackerson LM, Gomez V, et al. Effectiveness and reach of the FLU-FIT program in an integrated health care system: a multisite randomized trial. Am J Public Health 2013;103(6):1128–33.

52. Gupta S, Halm EA, Rockey DC, et al. Comparative effectiveness of fecal immunochemical test outreach, colonoscopy outreach, and usual care for boosting colorectal cancer screening among the underserved: a randomized clinical trial. JAMA Intern Med 2013;173(18):1725–32.

53. Church TR, Yeazel MW, Jones RM, et al. A randomized trial of direct mailing of fecal occult blood tests to increase colorectal cancer screening. J Natl Cancer Inst 2004;96(10):770–80.

54. Kempe KL, Shetterly SM, France EK, et al. Automated phone and mail population outreach to promote colorectal cancer screening. Am J Manag Care 2012;18(7): 370–8.

55. Levy BT, Daly JM, Xu Y, et al. Mailed fecal immunochemical tests plus educational materials to improve colon cancer screening rates in Iowa Research Network (IRENE) practices. J Am Board Fam Med 2012;25(1):73–82.

56. Liang PS, Wheat CL, Abhat A, et al. Adherence to competing strategies for colorectal cancer screening over 3 years. Am J Gastroenterol 2016;111(1):105–14.

57. Baker DW, Brown T, Buchanan DR, et al. Comparative effectiveness of a multifaceted intervention to improve adherence to annual colorectal cancer screening in community health centers. JAMA Intern Med 2014;174:1235–41.

58. Raich PC, Whitley EM, Thorland W, et al, Denver Patient Navigation Research Physicians. Patient navigation improves cancer diagnostic resolution: an individually randomized clinical trial in an underserved population. Cancer Epidemiol Biomarkers Prev 2012;21(10):1629–38.

59. Myers RE, Turner B, Weinberg D, et al. Impact of a physician-oriented intervention on follow-up in colorectal cancer screening. Prev Med 2004;38(4):375–81.

60. Arsenault PR, John LS, O'Brien LM. The use of the whole primary-care team, including community health workers, to achieve success in increasing colon cancer screening rate. J Healthc Qual 2016;38(2):76–83.

61. Kruse GR, Khan SM, Zaslavsky AM, et al. Overuse of colonoscopy for colorectal cancer screening and surveillance. J Gen Intern Med 2015;30(3):277–83.

62. Goodwin JS, Singh A, Reddy N, et al. Overuse of screening colonoscopy in the Medicare population. Arch Intern Med 2011;171(15):1335–43.

63. Yabroff KR, Klabunde CN, Yuan G, et al. Are physicians' recommendations for colorectal cancer screening guideline-consistent? J Gen Intern Med 2011; 26(2):177–84.

64. Gross CP, Andersen MS, Krumholz HM, et al. Relation between Medicare screening reimbursement and stage at diagnosis for older patients with colon cancer. J Am Med Assoc 2006;296(23):2815–22.

65. Ko CW, Sonnenberg A. Comparing risks and benefits of colorectal cancer screening in elderly patients. Gastroenterology 2005;129(4):1163–70.

66. Bibbins-Domingo K, U.S. Preventive Services Task Force. Aspirin use for the primary prevention of cardiovascular disease and colorectal cancer: U.S. Preventive Services Task Force recommendation statement. Ann Intern Med 2016; 164(12):836–45.

67. Kushi LH, Doyle C, McCullough M, et al. American Cancer Society Guidelines on nutrition and physical activity for cancer prevention: reducing the risk of cancer with healthy food choices and physical activity. CA Cancer J Clin 2012;62(1): 30–67.

Lung Cancer Screening

Richard M. Hoffman, MD, MPH[a],*, Rolando Sanchez, MD[b]

KEYWORDS

- Lung neoplasms • Early detection of cancer • Practice guidelines • Decision making
- Tomography, X-ray computed • Tobacco use

KEY POINTS

- Lung cancer is the leading cause of cancer death in the United States (US).
- More than 80% of lung cancer deaths are attributed to tobacco use highlighting the importance of primary prevention.
- A US trial showed that screening high-risk patients with low-dose computed tomography scans reduced lung cancer mortality by 20% compared with chest radiography.
- The US Preventive Services Task Force recommends annual lung cancer screening for high-risk patients (30 pack-years, current or quit within 15 years) aged 55 to 80 years.
- The Centers for Medicare and Medicaid will cover screening but requires programs to engage patients in shared decision-making, offer smoking cessation, and report data to a central registry.

INTRODUCTION

Lung cancer is the second most frequently diagnosed cancer in the United States and the leading cause of cancer death. In 2016, 224,390 new lung cancer cases were expected along with 158,080 lung cancer–related deaths.[1] More than 80% of these deaths are attributable to tobacco exposure making primary prevention the most effective cancer control strategy.[2] Although the 5-year survival for early stage lung cancers exceeds 50%, most cancers are detected at advanced stage when survival is poor.[3] Consequently, screening has been proposed as a strategy for reducing lung cancer mortality. Controlled trials have shown chest radiography and sputum cytology to be ineffective screening tests,[4] but screening with low-dose computed tomography (LDCT) can significantly reduce lung cancer mortality.[5]

This review focuses on the LDCT screening trials, particularly the National Lung Screening Trial (NLST), the subsequently issued screening guidelines, and challenges

Disclosure Statement: Neither author has any financial interests to disclose for this article.
[a] Department of Medicine, University of Iowa Carver College of Medicine, 200 Hawkins Drive SE 618 GH, Iowa City, IA 52242, USA; [b] Department of Medicine, University of Iowa Carver College of Medicine, 200 Hawkins Drive C325 GH, Iowa City, IA 52242, USA
* Corresponding author.
E-mail address: Richard-m-Hoffman@uiowa.edu

Med Clin N Am 101 (2017) 769–785
http://dx.doi.org/10.1016/j.mcna.2017.03.008
0025-7125/17/Published by Elsevier Inc.

medical.theclinics.com

and strategies for implementing screening programs in community practice. The review begins by briefly discussing the clinical presentation, pathology, staging, treatment options, survival, and primary prevention strategies for lung cancer.

CLINICAL PRESENTATION

Patients with early stage lung cancers are usually asymptomatic, presenting with lung nodules or a mass discovered incidentally on a chest radiograph or computed tomography (CT) scan. The clinical presentation with advanced disease is mostly related to the local tumor invasion, regional spread, distant metastasis, and paraneoplastic syndromes. These patients most commonly present with cough (50%–75%), hemoptysis (25%–50%), dyspnea (25%), and chest pain (20%).[6]

PATHOLOGY

Although recent guidelines emphasize immunohistochemical categories,[7] lung cancers have traditionally been classified histologically as small cell lung cancer (SCLC) or non–SCLC, with the latter group including adenocarcinoma, squamous cell carcinoma, and large cell carcinoma. Recent data from the Surveillance, Epidemiology, and End Results Program (SEER) registry show that adenocarcinoma (45%), squamous cell carcinoma (23%), and small cell carcinoma (13%) account for most US lung cancers.[3]

STAGING

Lung cancer is staged with the Tumor Node Metastasis (TNM) system.[8] The TNM system is also used for SCLC, though 90% of patients with these cancers present with advanced disease.

TREATMENT OPTIONS

Patients with early stage NSCLC and no contraindications for surgery should undergo surgical resection.[9] Nonsurgical candidates can be offered stereotactic body radiation therapy or radiofrequency ablation. Patients with early stage cancers with high-risk features or those with ipsilateral nodal involvement should receive adjuvant chemotherapy. Patients with SCLC and clinically limited stage are candidates for curative-intent chemoradiation.[10] Treatment recommendations for more advanced-stage cancers are beyond the scope of this review.

SURVIVAL

The overall average 5-year survival of US patients with lung cancer is 17.7%; however, survival varies markedly by stage at diagnosis (**Fig. 1**).[3] The average 5-year survival for patients with localized disease is 55.2%, though only 16.0% of patients are diagnosed at this stage.

CANCER CONTROL STRATEGIES
Primary Prevention

Smoking prevention and cessation are the best strategies for reducing lung cancer mortality and all deaths due to tobacco-related diseases.[11,12] Pharmacotherapy and behavioral interventions can help patients quit smoking.[13] However, as the prevalence of tobacco smoking continues to decrease, the incidence of lung cancer among non-smokers seems to be increasing.[14] This finding has prompted strategies to mitigate

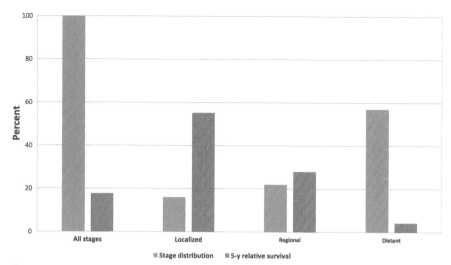

Fig. 1. Lung cancer stage distribution and survival, SEER Cancer Statistics Review, 2006 to 2012.

environmental and occupational exposure to carcinogens, including second-hand smoke, radon, asbestos, arsenic, metals, fiber, dust, organic compounds, and air pollution.[15] The efficacy of these interventions in reducing lung cancer mortality is unknown.

Secondary Prevention (Screening)

Chest radiography and sputum cytology
These tests are not recommended for lung cancer screening, either alone or in combination, because there is no evidence that they reduce lung cancer mortality.[4]

Low-dose computed tomography
The NLST, which published results in 2011, demonstrated a mortality benefit for screening high-risk individuals with LDCT lung scans (**Table 1**).[16] The NLST enrolled 53,454 participants at 33 medical centers in the United States. Participants were ever smokers aged 55 to 74 years, with a minimum 30-pack-year history of tobacco smoking who were currently smoking or had quit within the past 15 years. The NLST randomly assigned participants to undergo 3 rounds of annual screenings with LDCT or chest radiography.

The LDCT group had more lung cancer diagnoses than the radiography group (1060 vs 941) and a higher proportion of lung cancers detected at stage I or II (70.0% vs 56.7%). After a median 6.5 years of follow-up, lung cancer mortality was 20% lower in the LDCT group compared with the radiography group, with an absolute risk reduction of 0.3 percentage points (1.3% vs 1.6%). The number needed to screen with 3 rounds of LDCT to prevent one death from lung cancer was 320. Subgroup analyses suggest that women and blacks might have the greatest lung cancer mortality benefit.[17,18] Overall mortality was reduced by 6.7% in the LDCT group.

European LDCT screening trials have not shown a decrease in lung cancer mortality (see **Table 1**).[19–22] However, these trials differed from the NLST in having smaller sample sizes, enrolling a lower-risk cohort, and in the strategies used for managing pulmonary nodules. The Dutch-Belgian Randomized Lung Cancer Screening Trial

Table 1
Comparison of randomized controlled trials evaluating low-dose computed tomography screening for lung cancer

	NLST[16]	DANTE[19]	DLCST[20]	MILD[21]	NELSON[73]
Population features	United States Aged 55–74 y Men and women Smoking history: ≥30 pack-y Quit ≤15 y	Italy Ages 60–74 y Men only Smoking history: ≥20 pack-y Quit ≤10 y	Denmark Aged 50–70 y Men and women Smoking history: ≥20 pack-y Quit ≤10 y	Italy Aged 55–74 y Men and women Smoking history: ≥30 pack-y Quit ≤15 y	Netherlands/Belgium Aged 50–75 y Men and women Smoking history: ≥15 pack-y Quit ≤10 y
Study arms: number of participants	LDCT: 26,722 CXR: 26,732	LDCT: 1264 CXR + sputum cytology: 1186	LDCT: 2052 No screening: 2052	LDCT (annual): 1190 LDCT (biennial): 1186 No screening: 1723	LDCT: 7915 No screening: 7907
Statistical power	90% power to detect 21% reduction in lung cancer mortality	Unpowered	Unpowered	Unpowered	80% power to detect 20%–25% reduction in lung cancer mortality
Median follow-up	6.5 y	8.35 y	9.8 person-y	4.4 y	Ongoing (target: 10 y)
Lung cancer mortality rate (per 100,000 person-y), risk	LDCT: 247 Control: 309 PP = 0.80; 95% CI: 0.73–0.93	LDCT: 543 Control: 544 HR = 0.99; 95% CI: 0.69–1.43	LDCT: 200 Control: 190 HR = 1.03; 95% CI: 0.66–1.6	LDCT (annual): 216 LDCT (biennial): 109 Control: 109 HR = 1.52; 95% CI: 0.63–3.65	Not available
Absolute lung cancer mortality and risk reduction	LDCT: 1.3% Control: 1.6% ARR = 0.3 percentage points	LDCT: 4.7% Control: 4.6% ARI = 0.03 percentage points	LDCT: 1.90% Control: 1.85% ARI = 0.05 percentage points	LDCT (total): 0.76% Control: 0.41% ARI = 0.35 percentage points	Not available

Abbreviations: ARI, absolute risk increase; ARR, absolute risk reduction; CI, confidence interval; CXR, chest radiograph; DANTE, detection and screening of early lung cancer by novel imaging technology and molecular essays; DLCST, Danish Lung Cancer Screening Trial; HR, hazard ratio; MILD, Multicentric Italian Lung Detection; NELSON, Nederlands Leuvens Longkanker Screenings Onderzoek; NLST, National Lung Screening Trial; PP, percentage points.

(Nederlands Leuvens Longkanker Screenings Onderzoek [NELSON] trial) is an ongoing randomized controlled trial evaluating LDCT.[23,24] NELSON has enrolled nearly 16,000 ever smokers aged 50 to 75 years, including 5-year lung cancer survivors, and randomized them to LDCT at increasing screening intervals (1, 2, and 2.5 years) versus no screening. NELSON will assess survival, quality of life, smoking cessation, and cost-effectiveness.

SCREENING GUIDELINES

In early 2014, the US Preventive Services Task Force (USPSTF) gave a B recommendation to LDCT screening, implying moderate certainty of at least moderate net benefit.[25] The recommendation was based on microsimulation modeling[26] calibrated to data from the NLST and the Prostate, Lung, Colorectal, and Ovarian Cancer Screening Trial.[27] The simulated target population was a 100,000-person US cohort born in 1950 and followed from 45 to 90 years of age. The best-case scenario was to screen annually those meeting NLST smoking criteria from 55 through 80 years of age. This scenario was estimated to detect 50% of cancers at an early stage, reduce lung cancer mortality by 14% (number needed to screen of 575), and avert 497 lung cancer deaths (average gain of 10.6 life-years per death averted). Harms included 67,550 false-positive test results, 910 invasive diagnostic procedures for benign lesions, and 190 (9.9%) overdiagnoses among cases of screen-detected lung cancers. Radiation exposure resulted in 24 deaths.

Other professional societies also endorsed LDCT screening (**Table 2**), including the American Association for Thoracic Surgery (ATTS),[28] the American Cancer Society,[29] the American College of Chest Physicians, American Society of Clinical Oncology,[30,31] the American Lung Association,[32] the American Thoracic Society,[33] and the National Comprehensive Cancer Network (NCCN).[34] Although these guidelines routinely advised screening patients meeting NLST eligibility criteria, the ATTS and NCCN also recommended screening persons at 50 years of age with a 20 pack-year or greater smoking history if they had a cumulative 5-year cancer incidence risk of 5% or greater (ATTS) or an additional risk factor for lung cancer (NCCN). However, some experts cautioned against screening patients not meeting NLST criteria given the uncertainty about the balance of benefits and harms.[29,31]

Several important messages emerged across the guidelines. One was that patients should have access to high-quality, high-volume centers similar to those enrolling patients in the NLST. Screening is also not considered appropriate for those with substantial comorbidity, such as severe emphysema or cardiovascular disease, that would preclude attempting curative therapy or limit life expectancy. Lung cancer screening does not replace smoking cessation, and screening programs should provide support for smoking cessation and preventing relapse. The absolute benefit of screening is small, and the proportion of false-positive results is high; there are potential harms associated with invasive diagnostic procedures, radiation exposure, and incidental findings. Guidelines encourage providers to ensure that patients are making informed decisions.

The Centers for Medicare and Medicaid Services (CMS) issued a National Coverage Determination in early 2015 supporting annual lung cancer screening with LDCT.[35] Appropriate beneficiaries are asymptomatic adults aged 55 to 77 years meeting NLST criteria for smoking history. However, CMS also issued stringent criteria for reimbursement, including confirmation that a beneficiary met eligibility criteria and had undergone a counseling and shared decision-making visit. CMS had further stipulations regarding the qualifications and experience of the radiologists, the technical

Table 2
Guideline recommendations for lung cancer screening

Organization	Eligibility		Frequency	Setting	Counseling
	Age (y)	Tobacco History			
USPSTF (2013)[25]	55–80	≥30 pack-y; currently smoking or quit within 15 y Screening might not be appropriate for those with substantial comorbidity	Annual	Clinical settings that have high rates of diagnostic accuracy, appropriate follow-up protocols for positive results, and clear criteria for invasive procedures	Shared decision-making for screening Smoking cessation
American Cancer Society (2013)[29]	55–74	≥30 pack-y; currently smoking or quit within 15 y Relatively good health	Annual	Organized screening program with expertise in screening and access to multidisciplinary team skilled in evaluating, diagnosing, and treating lung abnormalities	Informed and shared decision-making for screening Smoking cessation
American Thoracic Society (2015)[33]	55–74	≥30 pack-y; currently smoking or quit within 15 y	Annual	Clinical settings that have high rates of diagnostic accuracy, appropriate follow-up protocols for positive results, and clear criteria for invasive procedures	Shared decision-making to allow patients to weigh trade-offs based on their personal risk profiles and make informed decision whether to screen Integrate smoking abstinence efforts into screening programs
American Association of Thoracic Surgery (2012)[28]	55–79 50–79	≥30 pack-y; ever smoker regardless of time since quitting 20 pack-y with risk factor (5-y risk ≥5%)	Annual	Environments where multidisciplinary teams are available for managing indeterminate and positive findings	Use risk calculators to determine high-risk population Support smoking cessation
National Comprehensive Cancer Network[34]	55–74 50–74	≥30 pack-y; currently smoking or quit within 15 y ≥20 pack-y; 1 additional risk factor[a]	Annual	Minimize screening risk by algorithmic management and multidisciplinary expertise	Shared decision-making to include discussion of benefits and risks
American College of Chest Physicians (2013)[31]	55–74	≥30 pack-y; currently smoking or quit within 15 y Suggest not screening those with severe comorbidity	Annual	Settings that can deliver the comprehensive care provided to NLST participants	Complete description of potential benefits and harms so that the individual can decide whether to undergo screening
American Lung Association (2015)[32]	55–74	≥30 pack-y; currently smoking or quit within 15 y	Annual	Link screening to accessing best practice multidisciplinary teams that can provide follow-up workup and care	Develop shared decision-making toolkits Provide smoking cessation services

[a] Cancer history, family history, disease history (chronic obstructive pulmonary disease, pulmonary fibrosis), occupational/environmental exposures (asbestos, radon, silica, and so forth).

specifications of the imaging modalities, and the use of a standardized lung nodule classification and reporting system.

SHARED DECISION-MAKING

The CMS requirement for shared decision-making was unprecedented for cancer screening but an explicit acknowledgment that these decisions are preference sensitive.[36] Shared decision-making is a process whereby patients and providers work together to make a health care decision based on the best available evidence and the patients' values and preferences.[37,38] CMS called for informing patients about the potential benefits and risks of screening, the diagnostic testing to evaluate positive screening results, the probability of false-positive tests, overdiagnosis, the total radiation exposure, the importance of adhering to annual screening, as well as the impact of patients' ability and/or willingness to undergo diagnosis and treatment on screening decisions.[35] Experts have suggested that these discussions also address tobacco harms other than lung cancer as well as strategies to avoid environmental and occupational risks for lung cancer.[39]

Using decision aids is a practical strategy for supporting shared decision-making. Decision aids are educational tools, which can be written, video, or Web-based, that should provide objective, balanced information about the options and potential outcomes, help elicit patients' values for these potential outcomes, and provide guidance for discussing screening decisions with a provider.[40] A Cochrane Collaboration review found that providing patients with decision aids for health treatment or screening decisions increased their engagement in decision-making, increased knowledge and improved the accuracy of risk perceptions, reduced decisional conflict, and increased the likelihood of making a values-congruent decision.[40] Several lung cancer screening decision aids are available (**Table 3**).

TRANSLATING RESEARCH INTO PRACTICE
Generalizability of National Lung Screening Trial

A criticism of the NLST was that participants were not representative of the general population. Less than 10% were members of minority populations; compared with the general population of tobacco users surveyed by the US Census Bureau's Tobacco Use Supplement meeting study eligibility criteria, NLST participants were younger, more likely to be former smokers, and of higher socioeconomic status.[5] The lack of representativeness is problematic because minorities and people of lower socioeconomic status are at a highest risk for dying of lung cancer.[41] Adherence to the screening protocol was 95% in the trial but might be considerably lower in community settings. Furthermore, most study sites were academic medical centers. Radiologists were experienced chest CT readers who underwent training for lung nodule interpretation. The overall complication rate for diagnostic procedures following a positive screening test was only 1.4%, and the 60-day operative mortality rate was just 1%. Although not derived from screening populations, previous Medicare data suggested substantially higher complication and mortality rates from invasive diagnostic procedures and lung resections.[42,43]

These issues were highlighted by the American Academy of Family Physicians (AAFP) who concluded that data were insufficient to recommend for or against LDCT screening.[44] The AAFP cited concerns about the unknown harms of expanding screening to community practice and extrapolating data from just 3 annual screens. The Medicare Evidence Development and Coverage Advisory Committee, convened by the CMS to review the evidence on lung cancer screening, expressed a lack of

Table 3
Lung cancer screening decision aids

Organization	Title	URL
Agency for Health Research and Quality	Lung Cancer Screening Tools for Patients and Clinicians	http://effectivehealthcare.ahrq.gov/index.cfm/tools-and-resources/patient-decision-aids/lung-cancer-screening/
American Thoracic Society	Decision Aid for Lung Cancer Screening with Computerized Tomography (CT)	https://www.thoracic.org/patients/patient-resources/resources/decision-aid-lcs.pdf
University of Michigan	Lung Cancer CT Screening: Should I get screened?	http://www.shouldiscreen.com
Memorial Sloan Kettering Cancer Center	Lung Cancer Screening Decision Tool	https://www.mskcc.org/cancer-care/types/lung/screening/lung-screening-decision-tool
The Dartmouth Institute	Option Grid decision aid: Lung cancer screening: yes or no?	http://optiongrid.org/option-grids/grid-landing/8
National Cancer Institute	Patient and Physician Guide: NLST	https://www.cancer.gov/types/lung/research/NLSTstudyGuidePatientsPhysicians.pdf
US Department of Veterans Affairs	Screening for Lung Cancer	http://www.prevention.va.gov/preventing_diseases/screening_for_lung_cancer.asp
NCCN	Lung Cancer Screening	https://www.nccn.org/patients/guidelines/lung_screening/#20

confidence that lung cancer screening could be effectively and safely performed in the Medicare population.[45] Meanwhile, they strongly thought that a clinically significant evidence gap remained regarding LDCT screening in the Medicare population outside a clinical trial.

Guidelines have explicitly addressed these concerns, advising that patients undergo screening only in qualified centers. The CMS recommendations also specified that screening centers contribute data to a certified national registry. Data elements include abnormal findings, diagnostic evaluations, cancer diagnoses, and treatments. Registry data will provide population-based data on practice patterns and outcomes that will help evaluate the effectiveness and safety of translating clinical trial results to community practice. Currently the American College of Radiology (ACR) hosts the only certified registry.[46]

Potential Harms

False-positive results

In the NLST, 26% of all LDCT screening tests were positive and nearly 40% of all participants had at least one positive result.[16] However, 96.4% of the positive screening results were false positives. NLST radiologists used a 4-mm threshold to characterize nodules as abnormal. The ACR has subsequently developed the Lung Imaging Reporting and Data System (Lung-RADS) classification scheme (**Table 4**), which defines suspicious solid nodules as being 8 mm or larger.[47] Investigators retrospectively applied Lung-RADS criteria to NLST images and found striking improvements in

Table 4
Summary of Lung Imaging Reporting and Data System classification for baseline screening

Category	Category Descriptor	Category	Findings	Management
Negative	No nodules and definitely benign nodules	1	No lung nodules Nodules with calcification	Continued annual screening with LDCT in 12 mo
Benign appearance or behavior	Nodules with a very low likelihood of becoming a clinically active cancer because of site or lack of growth	2	Solid/part solid nodules: <6 mm Ground-glass nodules: <20 mm	
Probably benign	Probably benign findings, short-term follow-up suggested; includes nodules with a low likelihood of becoming a clinically active cancer	3	Solid nodules: ≥6 to <8 mm at baseline OR new 4 mm to <6 mm Part solid nodules: ≥6 mm with solid component <6 mm Ground-glass nodules ≥20 mm	6-mo LDCT
Suspicious	Findings for which additional diagnostic testing and/or tissue sampling is recommended	4A	Solid nodules: ≥8 to <15 mm Part solid nodules: ≥8 mm with solid component ≥6 mm to <8 mm	3-mo LDCT; PET/CT may be used when there is a ≥8-mm solid component
		4B	Solid nodules: ≥15 mm Part solid nodules with solid component ≥8 mm	Chest CT with or without contrast, PET/CT and/or tissue sampling depending on the probability of malignancy and comorbidities
		4X	Category 3 or 4 nodules with additional features or imaging findings that increases the suspicion of malignancy	

specificity.[48] Applying Lung-RADS could have reduced the false-positive rate for baseline images from 26.6% to 12.8% and reduced the false-positive rate for follow-up examinations from 21.8% to 5.3%. The trade-off, though, was lower sensitivity: an 8.6 percentage point decrease for baseline images and a 15.2 percentage point decrease for follow-up images. The clinical consequences of potentially delaying cancer diagnoses are unknown.

Overdiagnosis

A recognized potential consequence of screening programs is overdiagnosis, that is, finding histologically confirmed cancers that would not have been otherwise diagnosed in the absence of screening. Based on measuring volume-doubling times to identify indolent cancers, an Italian observational study estimated the overdiagnosis rate to be about 25%.[49] A study modeling NLST data estimated an overall 18.5% probability of overdiagnosis with screening detection.[50]

Radiation exposure

The radiation exposure associated with low-dose CT scanning is about 1.5 mSv per examination.[30] In contrast, the radiation exposure is about 8 mSv from a diagnostic chest CT and up to 14 mSv from a PET/CT. Although calculations are based on indirect evidence, radiation exposure from LDCT lung cancer screening has been estimated to cause one cancer death for every 2500 screened subject over 20 years.[30] Some of this risk can be mitigated. CMS is requiring that screening centers confirm that patients are being exposed to low-dose radiation with screening chest CT scans. Applying Lung-RADS could help minimize radiation exposure from unnecessary diagnostic imaging. A retrospective analysis of NLST data also suggested that the screening interval might be lengthened following a normal baseline screen.[51]

Smoking Cessation

Lung cancer screening uniquely links diagnostic testing with an effective behavioral intervention: smoking cessation. NLST participants who were current smokers at the time of enrollment had more than a 2-fold increased lung cancer mortality during follow-up compared with former smokers, regardless of their screening arm.[52] Former smokers in the chest radiography screening arm who remained abstinent for 7 years had a 20% mortality reduction compared with current smokers, the same magnitude of benefit achieved with LDCT screening.

Lung cancer screening has been seen as a teachable moment when smokers are more susceptible to health messages about cessation and abstinence.[53] However, controlled screening trials have shown that screening alone will not affect smoking habits.[54–56] In contrast, abnormal LDCT findings are associated with smoking cessation.[56] NLST participants with nodules suspicious for lung cancer, particularly findings that were new or changed from a previous examination, were significantly less likely to continue smoking than participants with normal screening examinations (odds ratio = 0.66 [95% confidence interval (CI) 0.61–0.72]).[57] A clinical guideline from the Association for Treatment of Tobacco Use and Dependence and the Society for Research on Nicotine and Tobacco suggests that all smokers undergoing screening should be provided with evidence-based smoking cessation interventions.[58]

Cost-effectiveness

An estimated 7 million Americans would be eligible for lung cancer screening based on USPSTF screening criteria.[25] The total costs associated with screening could be substantial, potentially incurring $6.8 billion in Medicare expenditures over a 5-year time horizon.[59] However, analyses do suggest that lung cancer screening could provide good to moderate value.[60-62] One study based on NLST data estimated that the cost-effectiveness of screening would be $81,000 (95% CI 53,000–186,000) per quality-adjusted life-year.[60] However, estimates varied substantially by subgroups (**Table 5**).

Screening was much more cost-effective in NLST participants at higher risk for dying of lung cancer. A post hoc modeling study stratified this risk based on demographic and clinical risk factors and found that participants in the highest 3 quintiles of lung-cancer mortality risk accounted for 88% of the mortality benefit from screening.[63] Other investigators have developed risk calculators to predict lung cancer incidence to efficiently identify the ever smokers most likely to benefit from lung cancer screening.[64-66] **Box 1** shows some of the variables included in risk models. A prospective comparative analysis found that numerous lung cancer risk models more efficiently identified high-risk patients than the clinical trial eligibility criteria.[67] The best performing model, using a 6-year lung-cancer risk threshold of 0.0151 or greater, could reduce the number needed to screen to prevent one lung cancer death from the 320 in NLST to 255.[66] Applying risk calculators to identify the highest-risk patients, thus, could make screening more cost-effective. Applying Lung-RADS criteria that increase the threshold for classifying a nodule as abnormal and applying risk models to guide biopsy decisions[68] could also make screening more cost-effective as would successfully leveraging screening to increase smoking cessation and maintain abstinence.[62]

IMPLEMENTING LUNG CANCER SCREENING PROGRAMS
Recommendations

The American College of Chest Physicians and American Thoracic Society's policy statement on lung cancer screening identified crucial components for establishing a screening program (**Table 6**).[69] Speakers at a lung cancer screening workshop hosted by the National Academies of Sciences, Engineering, and Medicine highlighted the importance of creating a coordinated multidisciplinary team to address screening,

Table 5
Incremental cost-effectiveness lung cancer screening by National Lung Screening Trial subgroup

Characteristics		Number of Participants	Incremental Costs ($)	Incremental QALYs	Cost per QALY ($)
Sex	Male	31,446	1683	0.0115	147,000
	Female	21,856	1557	0.0340	46,000
Age at entry (y)	55–59	22,773	1541	0.0101	152,000
	60–64	16,333	1520	0.0320	48,000
	65–69	9504	1900	0.0351	54,000
	70–74	4685	1905	0.0163	117,000
Smoking status	Former	27,643	1661	0.0027	615,000
	Current	25,659	1601	0.0369	43,000
Risk of lung cancer	First quintile	10,660	1453	0.0086	169,000
	Second quintile	10,661	1454	0.0118	123,000
	Third quintile	10,660	1651	0.0061	269,000
	Fourth quintile	10,661	1672	0.0515	32,000
	Fifth quintile	10,660	1851	0.0354	52,000

Abbreviation: QALY, quality-adjusted life year.

Data from Black WC, Gareen IF, Soneji SS, et al. Cost-effectiveness of CT screening in the National Lung Screening Trial. New Engl J Med 2014;371(19):1793–802.

Box 1
Variables used in risk models for identifying high-risk patients

- Age
- Race/ethnicity
- Sex
- Body mass index
- Education
- Smoking status (current/former)
- Cigarettes smoked per day
- Smoking pack-years
- Age at smoking cessation
- Duration of smoking cessation
- Asbestos exposure
- Personal history of emphysema
- Personal history of malignant tumor
- Family history of lung cancer

Data from Li K, Husing A, Sookthai D, et al. Selecting high-risk individuals for lung cancer screening: a prospective evaluation of existing risk models and eligibility criteria in the German EPIC cohort. Cancer Prev Res 2015;8(9):777–85.

Table 6
Components necessary for a high-quality screening program: American College of Chest Physicians and American Thoracic Society

Component	Explanation
Who is offered lung cancer screening	Use NLST criteria, risk calculator to identify eligible subjects
How often, and for how long, to screen	Follow NLST, USPSTF, CMS criteria
How the CT scan is performed	Perform LDCT scans based on technical specifications
Identifying lung nodules	Policy on size threshold to label positive screening test
Structured reporting of screening results	Use Lung-RADS
Lung nodule management algorithm	Determine criteria for performing diagnostic procedures and entering patients into surveillance
Smoking cessation	Integrate within screening program
Patient and provider education	Use standardized materials, provider education
Data collection	Annually report data on each component of screening program as well as cancers diagnosed to central data registry

Data from Mazzone P, Powell CA, Arenberg D, et al. Components necessary for high-quality lung cancer screening: American College of Chest Physicians and American Thoracic Society policy statement. Chest 2015;147(2):295–303.

diagnosis, treatment, and smoking cessation.[39] They also noted the importance of having the electronic health record be able to readily identify eligible subjects; provide templates for progress notes, order sets, and radiologic reports that comply with CMS standards; track abnormal results and follow-up; and transmit data to national registries.[39] Supporting meaningful shared decision-making may require involving advanced practice providers, nurses, trained navigators, or health coaches who can also support smoking cessation interventions. Programs have developed tool kits that include CMS criteria for lung cancer screening, decision aids, lists of ACR-accredited screening facilities, as well as overviews of insurance coverage issues.

Uptake

The uptake of lung cancer in clinical practice has been limited. A 2014 survey of screening centers identified by the Lung Cancer Alliance Screening Centers of Excellence database found 203 screening centers.[70] However, centers were not widely distributed; 11 states had no identified screening centers, and many states with high rates of lung cancer incidence and mortality had limited screening capacity, particularly in rural areas.[70] Additional concerns have been raised about having sufficient capacity for thoracic surgery.[71] Being able to provide widespread access to high-quality screening, diagnostic, and treatment centers will be essential to effectively and equitably implementing screening.

Future of Lung Cancer Screening

Guidelines and practices will likely evolve as more data become available on optimal strategies for selecting patients and managing abnormal images. Improvements in imaging and diagnostic techniques and treatments may make the screening process safer and more cost-effective. Expected decreases in smoking rates may reduce the number of people eligible for screening.[72] Regardless, screening will require substantial resources, so the budget impact and effectiveness of community-based programs will need ongoing evaluation.

REFERENCES

1. Siegel RL, Miller KD, Jemal A. Cancer statistics, 2016. CA Cancer J Clin 2016; 66(1):7–30.
2. U.S. Department of Health and Human Services. The health consequences of smoking: 50 years of progress. a report of the surgeon general. Atlanta (GA): U.S. Department of Health and Human Services; Centers for Disease Control and Prevention; National Cancers for Chronic Disease Prevention and Health Promotion; Office on Smoking and Health; 2014.
3. Howlader N, Noone AM, Krapcho M, et al. SEER cancer statistics review, 1975-2013. Bethesda (MD): National Cancer Institute; 2016.
4. Manser R, Lethaby A, Irving LB, et al. Screening for lung cancer. Cochrane Database Syst Rev 2013;(6):CD001991.
5. National Lung Screening Trial Research Team, Aberle DR, Adams AM, et al. Reduced lung-cancer mortality with low-dose computed tomographic screening. N Engl J Med 2011;365(5):395–409.
6. Kocher F, Hilbe W, Seeber A, et al. Longitudinal analysis of 2293 NSCLC patients: a comprehensive study from the TYROL registry. Lung Cancer 2015;87(2): 193–200.

7. Travis WD, Brambilla E, Nicholson AG, et al. The 2015 World Health Organization classification of lung tumors: impact of genetic, clinical and radiologic advances since the 2004 classification. J Thorac Oncol 2015;10(9):1243–60.

8. Edge SB, Compton CC. The American Joint Committee on Cancer: the 7th edition of the AJCC cancer staging manual and the future of TNM. Ann Surg Oncol 2010; 17(6):1471–4.

9. National Cancer Institute. Non-small cell lung cancer treatment (PDQ®). 2016. Available at: https://www.cancer.gov/types/lung/hp/non-small-cell-lung-treatment-pdq. Accessed April 1, 2017.

10. National Cancer Institute. Small cell lung cancer treatment (PDQ®). 2016. Available at: https://www.cancer.gov/types/lung/hp/small-cell-lung-treatment-pdq. Accessed April 1, 2017.

11. Jha P, Ramasundarahettige C, Landsman V, et al. 21st-century hazards of smoking and benefits of cessation in the United States. N Engl J Med 2013;368(4): 341–50.

12. Anthonisen NR, Skeans MA, Wise RA, et al. The effects of a smoking cessation intervention on 14.5-year mortality: a randomized clinical trial. Ann Intern Med 2005;142(4):233–9.

13. Stead LF, Koilpillai P, Fanshawe TR, et al. Combined pharmacotherapy and behavioural interventions for smoking cessation. Cochrane Database Syst Rev 2016;(3):CD008286.

14. Zell JA, Ou SH, Ziogas A, et al. Epidemiology of bronchioloalveolar carcinoma: improvement in survival after release of the 1999 WHO classification of lung tumors. J Clin Oncol 2005;23(33):8396–405.

15. Dela Cruz CS, Tanoue LT, Matthay RA. Lung cancer: epidemiology, etiology, and prevention. Clin Chest Med 2011;32(4):605–44.

16. National Lung Screening Trial Research Team, Aberle DR, Berg CD, et al. The National Lung Screening Trial: overview and study design. Radiology 2011;258(1): 243–53.

17. Pinsky PF, Church TR, Izmirlian G, et al. The National Lung Screening Trial: results stratified by demographics, smoking history, and lung cancer histology. Cancer 2013;119(22):3976–83.

18. Tanner NT, Gebregziabher M, Hughes Halbert C, et al. Racial differences in outcomes within the national lung screening trial. Implications for widespread implementation. Am J Respir Crit Care Med 2015;192(2):200–8.

19. Infante M, Cavuto S, Lutman FR, et al. Long-term follow-up results of the DANTE Trial, a randomized study of lung cancer screening with spiral computed tomography. Am J Respir Crit Care Med 2015;191(10):1166–75.

20. Wille MM, Dirksen A, Ashraf H, et al. Results of the randomized Danish lung cancer screening trial with focus on high-risk profiling. Am J Respir Crit Care Med 2016;193(5):542–51.

21. Pastorino U, Rossi M, Rosato V, et al. Annual or biennial CT screening versus observation in heavy smokers: 5-year results of the MILD trial. Eur J Cancer Prev 2012;21(3):308–15.

22. Becker N, Motsch E, Gross ML, et al. Randomized study on early detection of lung cancer with MSCT in Germany: results of the first 3 years of follow-up after randomization. J Thorac Oncol 2015;10(6):890–6.

23. Horeweg N, van Rosmalen J, Heuvelmans MA, et al. Lung cancer probability in patients with CT-detected pulmonary nodules: a prespecified analysis of data from the NELSON trial of low-dose CT screening. Lancet Oncol 2014;15(12): 1332–41.

24. van Iersel CA, de Koning HJ, Draisma G, et al. Risk-based selection from the general population in a screening trial: selection criteria, recruitment and power for the Dutch-Belgian randomised lung cancer multi-slice CT screening trial (NELSON). Int J Cancer 2007;120(4):868–74.

25. Moyer VA, U.S. Preventive Services Task Force. Screening for lung cancer: U.S. Preventive Services Task Force recommendation statement. Ann Intern Med 2014;160(5):330–8.

26. de Koning HJ, Meza R, Plevritis SK, et al. Benefits and harms of computed tomography lung cancer screening strategies: a comparative modeling study for the U.S. Preventive Services Task Force. Ann Intern Med 2014;160(5):311–20.

27. Oken MM, Hocking WG, Kvale PA, et al. Screening by chest radiograph and lung cancer mortality: the Prostate, Lung, Colorectal, and Ovarian (PLCO) randomized trial. JAMA 2011;306(17):1865–73.

28. Jaklitsch MT, Jacobson FL, Austin JH, et al. The American Association for Thoracic Surgery guidelines for lung cancer screening using low-dose computed tomography scans for lung cancer survivors and other high-risk groups. J Thorac Cardiovasc Surg 2012;144(1):33–8.

29. Wender R, Fontham ET, Barrera E Jr, et al. American Cancer Society lung cancer screening guidelines. CA Cancer J Clin 2013;63(2):107–17.

30. Bach PB, Mirkin JN, Oliver TK, et al. Benefits and harms of CT screening for lung cancer: a systematic review. JAMA 2012;307(22):2418–29.

31. Detterbeck FC, Mazzone PJ, Naidich DP, et al. Screening for lung cancer: diagnosis and management of lung cancer. 3rd ed: American College of Chest Physicians evidence-based clinical practice guidelines. Chest 2013;143(5 Suppl): e78S–92S.

32. Samet JM, Crowell R, Estepar RSJ, et al. Providing guidance on lung cancer screening to patients and physicians. Chicago (IL): American Lung Association; 2015.

33. Wiener RS, Gould MK, Arenberg DA, et al. An official American Thoracic Society/ American College of Chest Physicians policy statement: implementation of low-dose computed tomography lung cancer screening programs in clinical practice. Am J Respir Crit Care Med 2015;192(7):881–91.

34. Wood DE. National Comprehensive Cancer Network (NCCN) clinical practice guidelines for lung cancer screening. Thorac Surg Clin 2015;25(2):185–97.

35. Centers for Medicare & Medicaid Services. Decision memo for screening for lung cancer with low dose computed tomography (LDCT)(CAG-00439N). 2015. Available at: https://www.cms.gov/medicare-coverage-database/details/nca-decision-memo.aspx?NCAId=274. Accessed May 24, 2016.

36. Rimer BK, Briss PA, Zeller PK, et al. Informed decision making: what is its role in cancer screening? Cancer 2004;101(5 Suppl):1214–28.

37. Charles C, Gafni A, Whelan T. Shared decision-making in the medical encounter: what does it mean? (or it takes at least two to tango). Soc Sci Med 1997;44(5): 681–92.

38. Informed Medical Decisions Foundation. Why shared decision making? 2016. Available at: https://www.informedmedicaldecisions.org/shareddecisionmaking. aspx. Accessed April 1, 2017.

39. National Academies of Sciences, Engineering, and Medicine. Implementation of lung cancer screening: proceedings of a workshop. Washington, DC: The National Academies Press; 2016.

40. Stacey D, Legare F, Col NF, et al. Decision aids for people facing health treatment or screening decisions. Cochrane Database Syst Rev 2014;(1):CD001431.

41. Albano JD, Ward E, Jemal A, et al. Cancer mortality in the United States by education level and race. J Natl Cancer Inst 2007;99(18):1384–94.

42. Wiener RS, Schwartz LM, Woloshin S, et al. Population-based risk for complications after transthoracic needle lung biopsy of a pulmonary nodule: an analysis of discharge records. Ann Intern Med 2011;155(3):137–44.

43. Finlayson EV, Birkmeyer JD. Operative mortality with elective surgery in older adults. Eff Clin Pract 2001;4(4):172–7.

44. American Academy of Family Physicians. Lung cancer. 2013. Available at: http://www.aafp.org/patient-care/clinical-recommendations/all/lung-cancer.html. Accessed April 1, 2017.

45. Centers for Medicare & Medicaid Services. MEDCAC Meeting 4/30/2014-lung cancer screening with low dose computed tomography. 2014. Available at: https://www.cms.gov/medicare-coverage-database/details/medcac-meeting-details.aspx?MEDCACId=68. Accessed April 1, 2017.

46. American College of Radiology. Lung cancer screening registry. Available at: http://www.acr.org/quality-safety/national-radiology-data-registry/lung-cancer-screening-registry. Accessed April 1, 2017.

47. American College of Radiology. Lung CT screening reporting and data system (Lung-RADS). 2014. Available at: http://www.acr.org/~/media/ACR/Documents/PDF/QualitySafety/Resources/LungRADS/AssessmentCategories.pdf.

48. Pinsky PF, Gierada DS, Black W, et al. Performance of lung-RADS in the National Lung Screening Trial: a retrospective assessment. Ann Intern Med 2015;162(7):485–91.

49. Veronesi G, Maisonneuve P, Bellomi M, et al. Estimating overdiagnosis in low-dose computed tomography screening for lung cancer: a cohort study. Ann Intern Med 2012;157(11):776–84.

50. Patz EF Jr, Pinsky P, Gatsonis C, et al. Overdiagnosis in low-dose computed tomography screening for lung cancer. JAMA Intern Med 2014;174(2):269–74.

51. Patz EF Jr, Greco E, Gatsonis C, et al. Lung cancer incidence and mortality in National Lung Screening Trial participants who underwent low-dose CT prevalence screening: a retrospective cohort analysis of a randomised, multicentre, diagnostic screening trial. Lancet Oncol 2016;17(5):590–9.

52. Tanner NT, Kanodra NM, Gebregziabher M, et al. The association between smoking abstinence and mortality in the national lung screening trial. Am J Respir Crit Care Med 2016;193(5):534–41.

53. McBride CM, Emmons KM, Lipkus IM. Understanding the potential of teachable moments: the case of smoking cessation. Health Educ Res 2003;18(2):156–70.

54. Ashraf H, Saghir Z, Dirksen A, et al. Smoking habits in the randomised Danish Lung Cancer Screening Trial with low-dose CT: final results after a 5-year screening programme. Thorax 2014;69(6):574–9.

55. van der Aalst CM, van den Bergh KA, Willemsen MC, et al. Lung cancer screening and smoking abstinence: 2 year follow-up data from the Dutch-Belgian randomised controlled lung cancer screening trial. Thorax 2010;65(7):600–5.

56. Slatore CG, Baumann C, Pappas M, et al. Smoking behaviors among patients receiving computed tomography for lung cancer screening. Systematic review in support of the U.S. Preventive Services Task Force. Ann Am Thorac Soc 2014;11(4):619–27.

57. Tammemagi MC, Berg CD, Riley TL, et al. Impact of lung cancer screening results on smoking cessation. J Natl Cancer Inst 2014;106(6). dju084.

58. Fucito LM, Czabafy S, Hendricks PS, et al. Pairing smoking-cessation services with lung cancer screening: a clinical guideline from the association for the

treatment of tobacco use and dependence and the society for research on nicotine and tobacco. Cancer 2016;122(8):1150–9.

59. Roth JA, Sullivan SD, Goulart BH, et al. Projected clinical, resource use, and fiscal impacts of implementing low-dose computed tomography lung cancer screening in Medicare. J Oncol Pract 2015;11(4):267–72.

60. Black WC, Gareen IF, Soneji SS, et al. Cost-effectiveness of CT screening in the National Lung Screening Trial. N Engl J Med 2014;371(19):1793–802.

61. Pyenson BS, Henschke CI, Yankelevitz DF, et al. Offering lung cancer screening to high-risk Medicare beneficiaries saves lives and is cost-effective: an actuarial analysis. Am Health Drug Benefits 2014;7(5):272–82.

62. Villanti AC, Jiang Y, Abrams DB, et al. A cost-utility analysis of lung cancer screening and the additional benefits of incorporating smoking cessation interventions. PLoS One 2013;8(8):e71379.

63. Kovalchik SA, Tammemagi M, Berg CD, et al. Targeting of low-dose CT screening according to the risk of lung-cancer death. N Engl J Med 2013;369(3):245–54.

64. Bach PB, Kattan MW, Thornquist MD, et al. Variations in lung cancer risk among smokers. J Natl Cancer Inst 2003;95(6):470–8.

65. Katki HA, Kovalchik SA, Berg CD, et al. Development and validation of risk models to select ever-smokers for CT lung cancer screening. JAMA 2016; 315(21):2300–11.

66. Tammemagi MC, Church TR, Hocking WG, et al. Evaluation of the lung cancer risks at which to screen ever- and never-smokers: screening rules applied to the PLCO and NLST cohorts. PLoS Med 2014;11(12):e1001764.

67. Li K, Husing A, Sookthai D, et al. Selecting high-risk individuals for lung cancer screening: a prospective evaluation of existing risk models and eligibility criteria in the German EPIC cohort. Cancer Prev Res (Phila) 2015;8(9):777–85.

68. McWilliams A, Tammemagi MC, Mayo JR, et al. Probability of cancer in pulmonary nodules detected on first screening CT. N Engl J Med 2013;369(10):910–9.

69. Mazzone P, Powell CA, Arenberg D, et al. Components necessary for high-quality lung cancer screening: American College of Chest Physicians and American Thoracic Society policy statement. Chest 2015;147(2):295–303.

70. Eberth JM, Qiu R, Adams SA, et al. Lung cancer screening using low-dose CT: the current national landscape. Lung Cancer 2014;85(3):379–84.

71. Edwards JP, Datta I, Hunt JD, et al. The impact of computed tomographic screening for lung cancer on the thoracic surgery workforce. Ann Thorac Surg 2014;98(2):447–52.

72. Tramontano AC, Sheehan DF, McMahon PM, et al. Evaluating the impacts of screening and smoking cessation programmes on lung cancer in a high-burden region of the USA: a simulation modelling study. BMJ Open 2016;6(2). e010227.

73. Horeweg N, Scholten ET, de Jong PA, et al. Detection of lung cancer through low-dose CT screening (NELSON): a prespecified analysis of screening test performance and interval cancers. Lancet Oncol 2014;15(12):1342–50.

Prevention of Prostate Cancer Morbidity and Mortality
Primary Prevention and Early Detection

Michael J. Barry, MD, MACP*, Leigh H. Simmons, MD

KEYWORDS

- Prostate cancer • Prostate-specific antigen • Screening • Shared decision making

KEY POINTS

- More than any other cancer, prostate cancer screening with the prostate-specific antigen (PSA) test increases the risk a man will have to face a diagnosis of prostate cancer.
- The best evidence from screening trials suggests a small but finite benefit from prostate cancer screening in terms of prostate cancer–specific mortality, about 1 fewer prostate cancer death per 1000 men screened over 10 years.
- The more serious harms of prostate cancer screening, such as erectile dysfunction and incontinence, result from cancer treatment with surgery or radiation, particularly for men whose PSA-detected cancers were never destined to cause morbidity or mortality.
- Active surveillance has the potential to "uncouple" overdiagnosis from overtreatment.
- Because of the close balance of potential benefits and harms, informed men should have the opportunity to decide whether PSA screening is right for them.

INTRODUCTION: MAGNITUDE OF THE PROBLEM
Incidence and Mortality

Prostate cancer is an important health problem, with 181,000 new cases and 26,000 deaths predicted in the United States for 2016.[1] The estimated lifetime risk of a prostate cancer diagnosis is about 13%, whereas the risk of eventually dying of prostate

Disclosure: Dr M.J. Barry is President of the Informed Medical Decisions Foundation, a part of Healthwise, where he is also Chief Science Officer. Healthwise is a 501(c)3 nonprofit organization that produces and licenses educational and decision support materials. He is also a member of the United States Preventive Services Task Force (USPSTF). This article does not necessarily represent the views and policies of the USPSTF.
General Medicine Division, Massachusetts General Hospital, 50 Staniford Street, Suite 957, Boston, MA 02114, USA
* Corresponding author.
E-mail address: mbarry@partners.org

Med Clin N Am 101 (2017) 787–806
http://dx.doi.org/10.1016/j.mcna.2017.03.009
0025-7125/17/© 2017 Elsevier Inc. All rights reserved.

cancer is about 2.5%.[2] The median age at diagnosis is 66 years, and the median age at death is 80 years. The distribution of age at death is shown in **Fig. 1**.

Time Trends

With the introduction of the prostate-specific antigen (PSA) test in the late 1980s, prostate cancer incidence increased precipitously (**Fig. 2**). After peaking in 1992, incidence has fallen. Prostate cancer mortality increased and decreased similarly.[1] The age-adjusted prostate cancer death rates dropped from about 40 deaths per 100,000 men in 1992 to about 20 per 100,000 in 2013.[2] The latter figure is less than the baseline mortality of about 30 prostate cancer deaths per 100,000 men in the 1960s and 1970s, before the "PSA era." There is little debate that PSA screening led to the incidence peak in the early 1990s. However, more debate surrounds the subsequent decrease, which may be attributable to the depletion of cases among men being retested[3] as well a decrease in testing in response to clinical trial results and guidelines discouraging routine screening. Even more controversy surrounds the reasons for the mortality increase and decrease. The changes may be attributable to reduced mortality due to early detection, or improved treatment of both early- and late-stage prostate cancer. However, causation is hard to prove at the population level. Lung cancer mortality among men also peaked in the early 1990s and has fallen steadily since then, only coincidentally related to PSA testing.[1] Prostate cancer mortality has also fallen in the United Kingdom, despite little screening.[4] Other theoretic contributors include the introduction of statins for treatment of hypercholesterolemia,[5] with reports of positive effects on prostate cancer mortality in treatment trials.[6] However, analyses from screening trials have been less persuasive.[7]

Risk Factors

In addition to age and PSA testing, race and family history are the most important risk factors for prostate cancer. African American men have an age-adjusted incidence of about 200 per 100,000 men compared with 120 per 100,000 for white men. Differences

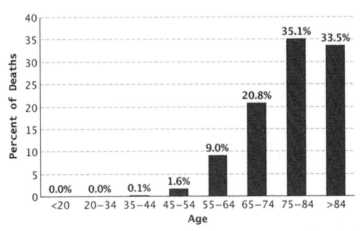

Fig. 1. Percent of prostate cancer deaths by age group, 2009-2013. (*Data from* Howlander N, Noone AM, Krapcho M, et al, editors. SEER cancer statistics review, 1975-2013. Bethesda (MD): National Cancer Institute. Available at: http://seer.cancer.gov/csr/1975_2013/. Based on November 2015 SEER data submission, posted to the SEER Web site. Accessed November 29, 2016.)

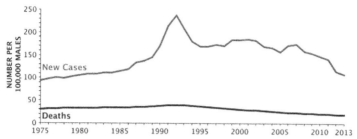

Fig. 2. US prostate cancer incidence and mortality, SEER 1975-2013, all races. Rates are age adjusted. (*Data from* Howlander N, Noone AM, Krapcho M, et al, editors. SEER cancer statistics review, 1975-2013. Bethesda (MD): National Cancer Institute. Available at: http:// seer.cancer.gov/csr/1975_2013/. Based on November 2015 SEER data submission, posted to the SEER Web site, April 2016.)

in death rates are even more dramatic, about 44 per 100,000 for African Americans, versus 19 per 100,000 for whites. Asians and Pacific Islanders, Native Americans, and Hispanic men all have a lower incidence of prostate cancer than whites, but only Asians and Pacific Islanders have appreciably lower mortalities, 9 per 100,000 versus 19 per 100,000 for whites. The lifetime risk of eventually dying of prostate cancer at age 50, when men might consider initiating screening, is about 4.7% for African Americans, 2.5% for whites, and 2.2% for Asians and Pacific Islanders.[2]

Men with a family history develop prostate cancer with a relative risk around 2.0.[8] A brother with prostate cancer is a stronger risk factor than a father. Quantifying the magnitude of the relationship between family history and prostate cancer incidence may be confounded by PSA testing, which is associated with both a positive family history and the risk of prostate cancer. Among cohorts of men routinely screened with PSA, a first-degree relative with prostate cancer was a weaker risk factor, with a relative risk of 1.3 to 1.6.[9,10] Little data are available on the effect of family history on prostate cancer mortality.

PRIMARY PREVENTION
Lifestyle and Nutrition

Epidemiologic observations that Asian men who assume a western diet have an increase in prostate cancer incidence have fueled interest in diet and lifestyle as modifiable risk factors. In a review of 176 meta-analyses addressing diet, body size, physical activity, and the risk of prostate cancer, no associations were graded with strong evidence.[11] A healthy diet and exercise are prudent for overall health, but cannot be strongly recommended for prostate cancer prevention.

Epidemiologic studies have raised interest in dietary supplements to lower prostate cancer risk.[12] Unfortunately, large randomized trials have not confirmed any benefit. The effect of 2 supplements was tested among more than 35,000 men in the Selenium and Vitamin E Cancer Prevention Trial. In this two-by-two factorial study, participants received either selenium (200 µg daily) or vitamin E (400 IU daily). Not only did selenium have no effect on prostate cancer incidence[13] but also, with extended follow-up, vitamin E supplementation was actually associated with a higher risk of prostate cancer.[14]

Chemoprevention

5-alpha-Reductase inhibitors (5-ARIs), like finasteride and dutasteride, reduce intra-prostatic levels of dihydrotestosterone. In theory, this reduction could reduce prostate cancer risk. This hypothesis was tested in the Prostate Cancer Prevention Trial (PCPT), where 18,882 men aged 55 or older with a normal digital rectal examination (DRE) and PSA level ≤3.0 ng/mL were randomized to finasteride 5 mg daily or placebo.[15] Men underwent prostate biopsies for cause during follow-up, and most underwent an end-of-study biopsy. Over 7 years, the incidence of prostate cancer was reduced from 24.4% with placebo to 18.4% with finasteride. Of note, even in the finasteride group, this cumulative incidence of prostate cancer was much higher than in the general population due to intensive surveillance in the trial. The reduced incidence of prostate cancer with finasteride was accompanied by a higher risk of sexual dysfunction, and of more concern, a significantly higher absolute risk of high-grade prostate cancer with finasteride versus placebo, 6.4% versus 5.1%.

Another trial compared dutasteride 0.5 mg daily with placebo among 6729 men with a baseline PSA of 2.5 to 10.0 ng/mL and a previous negative biopsy.[16] Men had rebiopsies at 2 and 4 years. Overall prostate cancer incidence decreased from 25.1% to 19.9% with dutasteride. However, in the third and fourth year of the study, 12 high-grade prostate cancers were diagnosed with dutasteride, compared with one with placebo.

A modeling study attempted to predict the impact on prostate cancer mortality from the data and suggested any mortality difference with a 5-ARI might be favorable or unfavorable.[17] Given the potential promotion of high-grade cancers, chemoprevention with 5-ARIs has not been widely embraced. A recent large nonexperimental study did not suggest a higher risk of prostate cancer death with 5-ARI use.[18]

THE PROSTATE-SPECIFIC ANTIGEN TEST

The PSA test was first approved by the US Food and Drug Administration (FDA) in 1986 for monitoring men with known prostate cancer. Clinicians quickly began to use the test for screening. An article by Catalona and colleagues[19] in 1991 is often cited as a sentinel publication in the dissemination of PSA screening, but incidence was already peaking by then (see **Fig. 2**). FDA approval of PSA for screening did not ensue until 1994. PSA is a protease made by prostatic epithelial cells that can be elevated in the setting of prostate cancer, but also in other prostate diseases, including benign prostatic hyperplasia, prostatic infection, and prostatic infarction (which may accompany acute urinary retention).[20] DREs do not appear to meaningfully increase PSA levels,[21] and only equivocal evidence supports an effect of long-distance bicycle riding or ejaculation.[22,23] Nevertheless, when repeating a mildly elevated PSA, avoidance of these factors may be reasonable. Antibiotic treatment of subclinical prostatitis in asymptomatic men with an elevated PSA without a documented infection is not recommended.[24]

Prostate-Specific Antigen Test Performance

The PSA test had disseminated widely before good data were available on test operating characteristics. The PCPT was the first large study to biopsy men regardless of PSA level, providing estimates of sensitivity and specificity. For men in the placebo arm, the traditional cut point of greater than 4.0 ng/mL was associated with about 20% sensitivity and 94% specificity for all cancers. For more important cancers with a Gleason grade of 7 or higher, and considering lower-grade cancers as noncancer, sensitivity was about 40% and specificity was 90%.[25] In terms of the "false reassurance rate," about 15% of men with a PSA level of 4.0 ng/mL or less had prostate cancer, and about 15% of those men had high-grade cancers.[26]

Risk Calculators

In general, the higher the PSA, the greater the risk of prostate cancer. However, data from the PCPT and other studies have shown that the slope of this relationship is flatter than previously thought, provoking controversy regarding what level of PSA should prompt a biopsy. The PCPT investigators have developed a risk calculator that can be used to help make informed decisions about biopsy.[27] Similar risk calculators have been developed from the European Randomized Study of Screening for Prostate Cancer (ERSPC; **Table 1**).[28]

Prostate-Specific Antigen Derivatives and Other Tests

An appreciation of the less-than-optimal performance of PSA has increased interest in "PSA derivatives," such as the percent free PSA, or rates of PSA change. Men with a lower percentage of circulating free PSA are more likely to have prostate cancer. However, only a relatively small percentage of men will have a high enough percent free PSA to mitigate against a biopsy.[29] A version of the PCPT risk calculator includes percent free PSA. A combination of total, free, and [−2]proPSA has been marketed to help make biopsy decisions among men with total PSA of 4 to 10 ng/mL. However, a negative test (at a cut point with 90% sensitivity for significant prostate cancer) is associated with a false reassurance rate of about 10%.[30] Other test combinations are being explored to improve specificity without sacrificing sensitivity.[31] Although an increasing PSA might seem a better predictor of prostate cancer than total PSA, analyses from multiple screening cohorts have not shown better performance of PSA "velocity" for discriminating men with and without prostate cancer, or for discriminating men with high-grade cancers from other men.[32–34] Men with a confirmed increase of ≥2.0 ng/mL in PSA level over 1 year may benefit from earlier consideration of biopsy, given that if they are diagnosed with prostate cancer, they have poorer outcomes with surgery.[35] Finally, treatment with a 5-ARI reduces PSA levels by about 50%.[36] To interpret PSA levels among adherent men, a reasonable recommendation is to double the value and interpret as usual.

THE DIGITAL RECTAL EXAMINATION

DREs are time-honored tests. DRE results can influence the likelihood of prostate cancer along with other predictors (see **Table 1**), and calculator estimates suggest slight increases in the risk of high-grade cancer even at low PSA levels with an abnormal

Table 1
Risk calculators for estimating the probability of prostate cancer at biopsy

Risk Calculator	Inputs	Outputs	URL
PCPTRC 2.0[27]	• Race • Age • PSA level • Family history • DRE result • Prior biopsy	Probability of: • High-grade cancer • Low-grade cancer • No cancer • Infection	http://deb.uthscsa.edu/ URORiskCalc/Pages/calcs.jsp
ERSPC Risk Calculator 4[a,28]	• DRE result • DRE volume • PSA level • Prior biopsy	Probability of: • Any cancer • High-grade or aggressive cancer	http://www.prostatecancer-riskcalculator.com/seven-prostate-cancer-risk-calculators

[a] Other ERSPC calculators are available at the same URL.

DRE. However, there is no direct evidence of an overall or disease-specific mortality benefit from DRE screening, and the ERSPC trial showing a benefit for screening did not include DRE (see next section).

THE EVIDENCE ON PROSTATE-SPECIFIC ANTIGEN SCREENING AND TREATMENT OF SCREEN-DETECTED CANCERS
Prostate, Lung, Colorectal and Ovarian Screening Trial

Randomized trials are the best way to determine whether a screening test reduces overall or disease-specific mortality as well as to define attributable harms. Two large screening trials dominate the evidence (**Table 2**). In the Prostate arm of the Prostate, Lung, Colorectal, and Ovarian Cancer Screening Trial (PLCO), about 77,000 men were recruited in 1993 to 2001 and randomized to screening with both PSA and DRE or "usual care." Men with a PSA level greater than 4 ng/mL or an abnormal DRE were referred back to their own clinicians, where relatively few underwent biopsy. Over 13 years of follow-up, the incidence of prostate cancer was significantly increased by 12% with screening, whereas prostate cancer mortality was not decreased.[37] The main critique of the PLCO trial has been that PSA screening was widespread in usual care in that era, and at least 50%, and possibly as many as 90%, of the men in the control group had at least one PSA test.[38] The PLCO investigators have described their study as a trial of "organized annual screening" versus "opportunistic screening."

To explore side effects of treatment of screen-detected cancers, the PLCO investigators matched prostate cancer survivors regardless of trial arm with noncancer controls. Regression analyses controlling for covariates revealed significantly poorer sexual and urinary function among the cancer survivors.[39]

European Randomized Study of Screening for Prostate Cancer Screening Trial

In the ERSPC trial, 162,243 men were randomized to screening with relatively infrequent PSA tests without DRE in 7 countries. A PSA greater than 3.0 ng/mL was generally considered positive. Although overall rates of contamination were not tracked, the 57% higher prostate cancer incidence with screening suggests relatively low rates of contamination compared with PLCO. In the ERSPC, the absolute reduction in prostate cancer mortality

Table 2
Major prostate-specific antigen screening trials

Screening Trial	Intervention	Screening Frequency	Duration (Last Report)	Incidence (per 10,000 Person-years) Control	Incidence (per 10,000 Person-years) Screen	Prostate Cancer Mortality (per 10,000 Person-years) Control	Prostate Cancer Mortality (per 10,000 Person-years) Screen
PLCO (US) Age 55–74 N = 76,685[37]	PSA DRE	Annual × 6 y Annual × 4 y	13 y (92% to 10 y, 57% to 13 y)	97.1 Relative risk (RR) 1.12 screening vs control (95% CI 1.07, 1.17)	108.4	3.4 RR 1.09 screening vs control (95% CI 0.87, 1.36)	3.7
ERSPC (Europe) Core age 55–69 N = 162,243[40]	PSA No DRE	Every 4 y (2 y in Sweden)	13 y	62.3 RR 1.57 screening vs control (95% CI 1.51, 1.62)	95.5	5.4 RR 0.79 screening vs control (95% CI 0.69, 0.91)	4.3

was a significant 1.1 fewer deaths per 10,000 person-years with screening in a "core" age group of men aged 55 to 69 years, or about 1 fewer prostate cancer death per 1000 men followed for 10 years. No benefit was seen in overall mortality.[40] In a subgroup analysis from 4 countries, screening also significantly reduced the cumulative incidence of metastases from 0.96% to 0.67% per 1000 men over 12 years.[41] Critiques of the ERSPC include heterogeneity of screening protocols and results among countries,[42] and different treatment patterns in the screening and control groups, although any impact of trial arm on treatment appears modest.[43,44] In an analysis of the increases in incidence and decreases in prostate cancer mortality by country, there was a strong positive relationship.[42] These findings imply that a greater mortality benefit comes at the price of more overdiagnosis and potentially overtreatment of screen-detected cancers.

Early results from the Rotterdam branch of the ERSPC showed that prostate biopsy was associated with relatively high rates of short-term pain (38%), hematuria (61%), rectal bleeding (25%), and hematospermia (62%).[45] However, overall quality of life and anxiety were not affected.[46] These results suggest the more serious harms of screening for prostate cancer are treatment-related side effects.

Other Data on Screening Harms

An even larger prospective study in the United Kingdom also examined the side effects of prostate biopsy. This study confirmed relatively high rates of short-term complications but also found increased anxiety among men with these complications.[47,48] Of note, large population-based studies have suggested a rising rate of infectious complications following biopsy requiring hospitalization; for example, about 7% in the Medicare population.[49]

Prostate Cancer Intervention Versus Observation Trial Treatment Trial

The Prostate Cancer Intervention Versus Observation Trial (PIVOT) recruited 731 men with clinically localized prostate cancer largely in Veterans Administration medical centers from 1994 to 2002 and randomized them to radical prostatectomy or observation, without intensive surveillance (**Table 3**).[50] About 20% of men assigned to radical prostatectomy did not ultimately undergo surgery, whereas about 20% randomized to observation eventually received attempted curative treatment. The primary endpoint was overall mortality, and about half of the men had died by the end of 10 years of follow-up. Neither overall nor prostate-cancer specific mortality was significantly lower with surgery. However, the risk of metastatic disease, often asymptomatic, was significantly reduced from 10.6% to 4.7%. Subgroup analyses suggested that men with higher-risk disease, as defined by a baseline PSA level greater than 10 ng/mL, or intermediate- or high-risk disease (taking into account PSA, and cancer grade, and stage) tended to benefit more from surgery.

In PIVOT, perioperative complications occurred in about 21% of men assigned to surgery, including one death. At 2 years of follow-up, about 17% of men randomized to surgery had urinary incontinence compared with 6% of men with observation; erectile dysfunction occurred in about 81% randomized to surgery versus 44% with observation.[50]

ProtecT Treatment Trial

The ProtecT trial in the United Kingdom enrolled 1643 men from 1999 to 2009, diagnosed with clinically localized prostate cancer in an organized PSA screening program (see **Table 3**). Participants were randomized to active monitoring (close surveillance with the intention to treat for evidence of progression), external beam radiotherapy with neoadjuvant androgen deprivation, or radical prostatectomy. Men enrolled in

Table 3
Major screen-detected prostate cancer treatment trials

Treatment Trial	Intervention	Duration	PCa Mortality			Overall Mortality		
			Obs/AS	RP	EBRT	Obs/AS	RP	EBRT
PIVOT (US) Mean age, 67 Median PSA, 7.8 ng/mL T1c, 51% N = 731[50]	Radical prosatectomy (RP) vs observation (Obs)	10 y median follow-up	21/364 (8.4%) HR 0.67 RP vs observation (95% CI .36, 1.09)	31/367 (5.8%)	—	183/367 (49.9%) HR 0.88 RP vs Obs (95% CI 0.71, 1.08)	171/364 (47.0%)	—
ProtecT (UK) Median age, 62 Median PSA, 4.6 ng/mL T1c, 76% N = 1643[51]	RP vs external beam radiotherapy (EBRT) vs active surveillance (AS)	10 y median follow-up	8/545 (1.4%) P = .48	5/553 (0.9%)	4/545 (0.7%)	59/545 (10.8%) P = .87	55/553 (9.9%)	55/545 (10.1%)

this trial were younger and healthier, with less advanced disease, than in PIVOT. There were no significant differences in prostate cancer–specific or overall mortality among the 3 arms. However, the cumulative incidence of metastatic disease, not always symptomatic, was significantly lower in the 2 active treatment arms, about 3% versus 6% with active monitoring. Moreover, over 10 years, about half the participants randomized to active monitoring eventually underwent treatment.[51]

Five-year data on patient-reported outcomes from ProtecT confirmed a persistent risk of sexual dysfunction and incontinence with surgery. Radiotherapy affected sexual and bowel function but not continence, and both sexual function and continence declined slowly with active monitoring. No significant differences were noted in measures of anxiety, depression, or overall quality of life.[52]

Modeling Studies to Extend the Results of the Screening Trials

Numerous studies have attempted to extend the results of screening trials to estimate benefits and harms under different conditions. For example, one study used data from the Rotterdam section of the ERSPC to estimate the effect of PSA screening on prostate cancer mortality correcting for the effects of nonattendance in the screening group and contamination in the control group. The relative risk estimate dropped from 0.68 to 0.49 with this correction, but with a higher risk of overdiagnosis.[53] Another group used 11-year results from ERSPC and utility assessments from the literature to quantify the impact of treatment side effects on quality of life. They found that side effects reduce the anticipated quality-adjusted life-years (QALYs) gained from screening 1000 men aged 55 to 69 from 73 to 56 in the base case, with considerable variability in the estimate depending on assumptions. In a microsimulation model, other investigators examined the implications of 35 different PSA screening strategies varying stop and start ages, screening intervals, and biopsy thresholds. In the base case with annual screening of men aged 50 to 74, they estimated the lifetime risk of prostate cancer death might drop from 2.86% to 2.15%, with an absolute risk of overdiagnosis of 3.3%. However, less frequent testing and higher biopsy thresholds for older men maintain most of the benefit with fewer false positives, albeit without much reduction in overdiagnosis.[54] This group also estimated the cost-effectiveness of 18 different screening strategies. They found that only screening with higher biopsy thresholds increased QALYs with contemporary treatment patterns, and only more selective treatment led to generally acceptable incremental cost-effectiveness ratios, from $71,000 to $136,000 per QALY.[55]

EVIDENCE-BASED UNITED STATES GUIDELINES ON PROSTATE CANCER SCREENING

Guidelines for prostate cancer screening have been issued by several organizations (**Table 4**).[56–61] The American College of Physicians (ACP) "guidance statement" was based on a review of other guidelines, whereas the others were based on formal systematic reviews. Both the US Preventive Services Task Force (USPSTF) and the American Society of Clinical Oncology (ASCO) used a systematic review developed for the Task Force[62]; The American Cancer Society (ACS) and the American Urological Association (AUA) conducted independent systematic reviews. Basically, the ACS, ACP, ASCO, and the AUA recommend a shared decision-making approach to individualize decisions about screening. Although the USPSTF recommended against PSA screening, judging that the benefits did not outweigh the harms, the recommendation acknowledged that shared decision making (SDM) should occur when the test is offered or requested. Of note, all 5 guidelines reviewed the same evidence, but

Table 4
Major, evidence-based guidelines for prostate cancer screening

Guideline	Most Recent Update	Key Recommendation Statement
ACS[56,57]	2010	"Men who have at least a 10-y life expectancy should have an opportunity to make an informed decision with their health care provider about whether to be screened for prostate cancer after receiving information about the potential benefits, risks, and uncertainties associated with prostate cancer screening; prostate cancer screening should not occur without an informed decision-making process."
ACP[58]	2013	ACP recommends that clinicians inform men between the ages of 50 and 69 y about the limited potential benefits and substantial harms of screening for prostate cancer. ACP recommends that physicians base the decision to screen for prostate cancer using the PSA test on the risk for prostate cancer, a discussion of the benefits and harms of screening, the patient's general health and life expectancy, and patient preferences. ACP recommends that clinicians should not screen for prostate cancer using the PSA test in patients who do not express a clear preference for screening.
ASCO[59]	2012	"In men with a life expectancy >10 y, it is recommended that physicians discuss with their patients whether PSA testing for prostate cancer screening is appropriate for them. PSA testing may save lives but is associated with harms, including complications, from unnecessary biopsy, surgery, or radiation treatment."
AUA[60]	2013	"For men ages 55–69 y the Panel recognizes that the decision to undergo PSA screening involves weighing the benefits of preventing prostate cancer mortality in 1 man for every 1000 men screened over a decade against the known potential harms associated with screening and treatment. For this reason, the Panel strongly recommends shared decision-making for men age 55–69 y that are considering PSA screening, and proceeding based on a man's values and preferences."
USPSTF[61]	2012	"The US Preventive Services Task Force recommends against prostate-specific antigen (PSA)-based screening for prostate cancer (grade D recommendation)."

differed in terms of panel members' assessments of the tradeoff between possible benefits and harms.

The AUA guideline recommends against screening men under the age of 40 and discourages routine screening in average-risk men aged 40 to 54. The AUA guideline also recommends a screening frequency of every 2 years. All guidelines recommend against screening men greater than the age of 69 or in poor health, although the ACS guideline recommends not screening men with less than a 10-year life expectancy, which comes at about age 76 for men with average comorbidity. A recently published tool allows estimation of life expectancy by age, race, and comorbidity.[63] However, there is little direct evidence that the benefits of screening outweigh the harms even for healthy men over the age of 69. These guidelines do not address the question of the PSA threshold to recommend biopsy, nor do they contradict the common practice of considering a biopsy for PSA greater than 4.0 ng/mL.

NEWER STRATEGIES DESIGNED TO IMPROVE THE RATIO OF SCREENING BENEFITS TO HARMS

A major problem with PSA screening is overdetection and overtreatment of prostate cancers not destined to cause future morbidity and mortality. Less intensive screening strategies; higher thresholds for biopsy, including use of newer imaging modalities to guide prostate biopsies; and active surveillance for some cancers are all being considered to maintain most screening benefits while reducing harms.

Screening Strategies

In the ERSPC, screening intervals of between 2 and 4 years led to decreased prostate cancer mortality.[40] An analysis from the PLCO trial suggested screening intervals related to baseline PSA: every 5 years for PSA less than 1 ng/mL, 2 years for PSA 1.0 to 1.99 ng/mL, and annual for PSA greater than 2.0 ng/mL.[64] Recommendations for aging men who have had regular PSA tests to stop screening can be challenging.[65] However, recent studies can help guide discussion. Men may be comforted to know that if the PSA level is ≤ 1.0 ng/mL at age 60, the chance of eventually dying of prostate cancer is only about 0.2%[66]; whereas in another cohort, 0/154 men aged 75 to 80 with a PSA level less than 3.0 ng/mL eventually died of prostate cancer.[67] Recent evidence suggests rates of PSA screening in the United States have dropped among men 75 or older from about 200 tests per 1000 person-years in 2008 to 125 in 2013.[68]

Biopsy Strategies

Higher PSA thresholds for biopsies may decrease the risk of overdiagnosis. Age- and race-specific reference ranges have been considered to increase sensitivity among younger men and increase specificity among older men.[69,70] The concern about higher biopsy thresholds has been aggressive cancers "escaping from cure" if not detected at lower PSA levels, although the substantial absolute benefit with surgery for men with a baseline PSA level greater than 10 ng/mL in PIVOT challenges this assumption. Repeating PSA levels when initial results are just over the biopsy threshold may also help reduce overdiagnosis.[71]

Traditionally, prostate biopsies have been guided using transrectal ultrasound. There is growing interest in MRI to evaluate men who have an elevated PSA level and to direct biopsies; a recent study examined the performance of MRI compared with the PCPT risk calculator. The MRI outperformed the risk calculator in the detection of high-grade prostate cancer.[72] A recent meta-analysis suggested use of MRI might increase sensitivity of biopsy for high-risk cancers and decrease sensitivity for low-risk cancers.[73] However, if both MRI-directed and traditional systematic biopsies are performed, increased sensitivity will be accompanied by more overdiagnoses. MRI obviously increases the cost and complexity of screening for an as yet uncertain effect on the ratio of benefits to harms.

Active Surveillance

The harms of screening largely reflect the side effects of treatment with surgery or radiation. Men diagnosed with prostate cancers that were never destined to cause morbidity or mortality can only be harmed. The indolent natural history of many PSA-detected cancers has led to strategies of active surveillance for men with low-risk cancers. These strategies involve following men closely with PSA tests, DREs, and biopsies, with the goal of treating for evidence of progression. Long-term outcomes of active surveillance have been favorable,[74,75] and in the ProtecT trial, prostate cancer mortality was similar to the active treatment strategies at 10 years.

However, the 3% absolute increase in the risk of metastases at 10 years must be kept in mind.[51] Active surveillance for the roughly two-thirds of newly diagnosed men who would qualify for this strategy has the potential for uncoupling overdiagnosis and over-treatment.[76] Much research is addressing the refinement of criteria for active surveillance, including genetic markers[77] as well as how "active" active surveillance needs to be.[78] Recent data suggest active surveillance is being used to a growing extent.[79,80]

SHARED DECISION MAKING TO IMPROVE DECISION QUALITY

Given that all screening guidelines discuss SDM, it is important to understand the approach. SDM is a strategy to ensure that patients and clinicians are well informed about the potential benefits and harms of testing and treatment options, and that patients have the opportunity to communicate their values and preferences with regard to medical decisions with more than one reasonable option. With SDM, it is more likely that decisions will be of high quality, meaning that tests or treatments chosen reflect the considered preferences of well-informed patients and are then implemented.[81]

SHARED DECISION MAKING FOR PROSTATE CANCER SCREENING
Current State of Shared Decision Making for Prostate-Specific Antigen Screening

Many men undergo PSA testing routinely, in some cases because of the apparent simplicity of checking a simple blood test, often in concert with other routine laboratory tests and in part because of the complexity of the discussion. Precisely because of this complexity, SDM provides an appropriate pause for patients and clinicians to ensure that they are on the same page with a screening plan given the patient's clinical situation and health goals.

Most men do not have PSA conversations with their clinicians that adequately address the core elements of SDM.[82] In 2009, the National Survey of Medical Decisions queried 375 men who had undergone or discussed PSA testing in the prior 2 years. Although 70% of men reported a discussion about screening before testing, the conversations emphasized the benefits of testing much more often than the disadvantages. In addition, only 60% of men who reported a conversation about screening recalled being asked their preference. Knowledge testing about prostate cancer incidence, mortality, and PSA test accuracy found that 48% failed to answer any of the 3 questions correctly.[83]

What to Cover in a Shared Decision-Making Conversation?

An SDM conversation should include the following elements: (1) discussion of the nature of the decision at hand and the desire to have patient's participation; (2) review of testing options and expected outcomes, including potential benefits and potential harms; (3) assessment and clarification of patient's values and preferences; and (4) a decision and its implementation. A variety of frameworks exists for SDM conversations, including the SHARE Approach developed by the Agency for Healthcare Research and Quality and the Six Steps of SDM developed by the Informed Medical Decisions Foundation.[84,85] A conversation about prostate cancer screening could include the points in **Box 1**. The ACS, ACP, and ASCO guidelines also provide talking points (see **Table 4**).

When possible, natural frequencies should be used to discuss risks and benefits (eg, "If 1000 men do not have the PSA blood test, 5 of those 1000 men will die from prostate cancer in the next 10 years. If 1000 men do have the PSA test done, 1 of those deaths will be prevented, and 4 will not.")

An assessment of a patient's risk factors should be performed and discussed in context of what that experience means for him. Inquiry about the experience of seeing

---

Box 1
Suggested content of a prostate-specific antigen shared decision-making discussion between clinician and patient

1. The PSA blood test can be elevated due to prostate cancer or other benign prostate conditions.

2. Men can decide to have or not have the PSA test, and there is no one right answer for everyone.

3. Having the PSA test increases the chance a man will be diagnosed with prostate cancer.

4. A PSA test may find a prostate cancer earlier than if no test is done.

5. Having a PSA test appears to lower the risk of dying of prostate cancer, but it does not appear to impact on a man's overall risk of dying from all causes.

6. An elevated PSA level will lead to a referral to a urology specialist, and further testing may include repeat PSA testing, imaging tests such as MRI or ultrasound, and prostate biopsy. It is the biopsy that eventually makes the diagnosis of prostate cancer, not the PSA test.

7. Most men with an elevated PSA will not be diagnosed with a prostate cancer.

8. Some men with a "normal" PSA level *do* have prostate cancer.

9. DRE has not been proven to be a useful screening test for prostate cancer, although it is often done as part of a general physical examination.

10. Management choices if prostate cancer is diagnosed may include active surveillance (repeat blood tests, digital rectal examinations, and biopsies over time), surgical removal of the prostate, and radiation treatment.

11. Long-term side effects of prostate cancer treatments include incontinence and difficulty with erections.

---

one's family members or friends undergo treatment of prostate cancer, especially if the cancer was detected by screening, may be a useful starting point for conversation. Patients and physicians should have an initial detailed discussion about PSA testing, which can then be revisited in light of new evidence or changes in the patient's life expectancy.

Role of Decision Aids

Decision aids are tools designed to help patients engage with their clinicians and become more informed about the benefits and harms of possible treatment options. They are designed to supplement, not replace, the conversation a patient has with his clinician. Examples of PSA patient decision aids can be found at <https://decisionaid.ohri.ca/azlist.html>.

OUTCOMES OF SHARED DECISION MAKING FOR PROSTATE CANCER SCREENING
Systematic Review of Decision Aids for Prostate-Specific Antigen Screening

A 2014 *Cochrane Review* assessed the effects of decision aids on PSA screening decisions. The pooled relative risk for 13 trials comparing decision aids to usual care on actually getting a PSA test was 0.87 (95% confidence interval [CI] 0.77–0.98), a significant reduction.[86]

Case Study: Prostate-Specific Antigen Decision Aids in Primary Care Practices at Massachusetts General Hospital

In 2005, Massachusetts General Hospital (MGH) in Boston began to study the use of video and booklet decision aids in primary care practice. These decision aids addressed 40 commonly encountered medical topics, including cancer screening decisions (eg, prostate cancer and colon cancer). Decision aid distribution was paired with a clinician training program on using decision aids effectively; this training has been delivered to 165 clinicians, mostly primary care physicians.[87]

The PSA screening program was an early favorite of the prescribing clinicians, and it remains one of the most frequently prescribed decision aids. In most cases, patients received the video program following their visit; however, in some practices, patients were sent the video program before a visit. A survey of 542 patients indicated the programs were highly rated (72% very good or excellent), and 87% stated that it was very or extremely important that clinicians provide such programs. Patients also scored highly on a 5-question test of their PSA knowledge (86% correct) after viewing the decision aid (Gerstein B, Stringfellow V. Primary care pre-/post-viewing data summary, Massachusetts General Hospital. Unpublished data, 2008).[88]

Informed Choices About Prostate-Specific Antigen Testing at Massachusetts General Hospital and Dartmouth Hitchcock Medical Center

The Informed Medical Decisions Foundation sponsored a large study of use of a video decision aid on PSA testing at Dartmouth Hitchcock Medical Center and MGH. These sites surveyed 3895 men before and after they viewed a 31-minute video decision aid, "The PSA Test: Is It Right for You?," that featured interviews with men who discussed how they reached their decisions about PSA testing. At one site, most of the decision aids were sent to men before a routine visit with primary care physicians. At the second site, clinicians prescribed the decision aid at the visit and patients watched it after the visit. Patients were surveyed beforehand to assess their leanings about PSA testing, readiness to decide, and their preferred role in decision making. Patients then watched the decision aid and completed a second questionnaire immediately, including the same initial items, as well as knowledge questions about the PSA screening, and whether they planned to discuss PSA testing with their clinician.

A total of 1041 (27%) participants returned all questionnaires. Half of the participants were between 50 and 59 years of age, and half had had a prior PSA test. The differences seen in patients' leaning regarding testing was most striking among the 32% who identified themselves as not sure before viewing. After viewing the decision aid, 38% leaned toward PSA screening; 17% were not sure, and 44% leaned away from screening (**Fig. 3**). The number of participants who felt close to making a decision

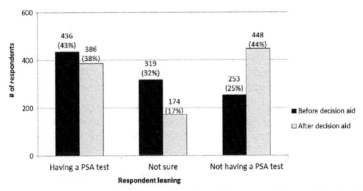

Fig. 3. PSA testing leanings reported by respondents before and after reading/viewing a decision aid (n = 1008 responding to both questions, $P<.001$, χ^2 test for overall changes in proportions across matched pairs).[89]

about PSA screening increased from 57% before viewing to 75% after viewing (P<.001). Also, men who answered more of the after viewing knowledge questions correctly were more likely to lean against screening.[89]

LEGAL ISSUES

Many physicians recall the upsetting 2004 essay by Dr Daniel Merenstein, who described his experience of meeting a patient once during his residency with whom he discussed the risks and benefits of PSA testing and documented that conversation. This patient was subsequently diagnosed with incurable prostate cancer, and Dr Merenstein and his training program were successfully sued for failing to practice the community standard of care, which was to order a PSA for men over the age of 50, without discussion.[90]

Since that time, greater lay understanding about the limited benefit and potential risks of PSA testing, as well as national guidelines recommending discussion, have tempered enthusiasm for testing men without conversations. A study by Barry and colleagues aimed to determine the impact of different strategies to document SDM about PSA by interviewing focus groups of potential jurors about a hypothetical case similar to the Merenstein case. Focus group participants felt that the documentation of a SDM conversation, and even better, the use of a decision aid to enhance the conversation, met the standard of care with regard to prostate cancer screening.[91]

SUMMARY AND CONCLUSIONS, RESEARCH NEEDS

Prostate cancer screening with the PSA test became widespread before the tradeoff between benefits and harms were clearly defined in clinical trials. As this evidence has accumulated, the balance between potential benefits and harms appears relatively close. Some men with aggressive prostate cancers likely benefit from early detection and treatment, whereas many more are harmed, largely by the side effects of treatment. Strategies are emerging that maintain most of the benefits of screening, while reducing the harms. At this point, sharing uncertainties with individual men through an SDM process may be the best way to resolve the PSA controversy, "one man at a time."[92]

More research is needed to develop testing strategies focused on diagnosing potentially fatal cancers at a point where treatment is still effective, while not detecting or at least not treating cancers not destined to cause future problems. More research is also needed to define practical implementation strategies to ensure all men have the opportunity to be informed and involved in the PSA decision to the extent they want to be.

REFERENCES

1. American Cancer Society. Cancer facts & figures 2016. Atlanta (GA): American Cancer Society; 2016.
2. Howlander N, Noone AM, Krapcho M, et al, editors. SEER cancer statistics review, 1975-2013. National Cancer Institute: Bethesda (MD). Available at: http://seer.cancer.gov/csr/1975_2013/. Based on November 2015 SEER data submission, posted to the SEER Web site. Accessed April 3, 2017.
3. Brawley OW. Prostate cancer epidemiology in the United States. World J Surg 2012;30(2):195–200.
4. Cancer Research UK. Prostate Cancer Statistics. Available at: http://www.cancerresearchuk.org/health-professional/cancer-statistics/statistics-by-cancer-type/prostate-cancer. Accessed November 29, 2016.

5. Gu Q, Paulose-Ram R, Burt VL, et al. Prescription cholesterol-lowering medication use in adults aged 40 and over: United States, 2003-2012. NCHS data brief, no. 177. Hyattsville (MD): National Center for Health Statistics; 2014.

6. Raval AD, Thakker D, Negri H, et al. Association between statins and clinical outcomes among men with prostate cancer: a systematic review and meta-analysis. Prostate Cancer Prostatic Dis 2016;19:151–62.

7. Platz EA, Tangen CM, Goodman PJ, et al. Statin drug use is not associated with prostate cancer risk in men who are regularly screened. J Urol 2014;192:379–84.

8. Bruner DW, Moore D, Parlanti A, et al. Relative risk of prostate cancer for men with affected relatives: systematic review and meta-analysis. Int J Cancer 2003;107:797–803.

9. Saarimaki L, Tammela TL, Maattanen L, et al. Family history in the finnish prostate cancer screening trial. Int J Cancer 2015;136:2172–7.

10. Randazzo M, Muller A, Carlsson S, et al. A positive family history as a risk factor for prostate cancer in a population-based study with organised prostate-specific antigen screening: results of the Swiss European Randomised study of Screening for Prostate Cancer (ERSPC, Aarau). BJU Int 2016;117:576–83.

11. Markozannes G, Tzoulaki I, Karli D, et al. Diet, body size, physical activity and risk of prostate cancer: an umbrella review of the evidence. Eur J Cancer 2016;69:61–9.

12. Poppel HV, Tombai B. Chemoprevention of prostate cancer with nutrients and supplements. Cancer Manag Res 2011;3:91–100.

13. Lippman SM, Klein EA, Goodman PJ, et al. The Selenium and Vitamin E Cancer Prevention Trial (SELECT). JAMA 2009;301:39–51.

14. Klein EA, Thompson IM, Tangen CM, et al. Vitamin E and the risk of prostate cancer: updated results of the Selenium and Vitamin E Cancer Prevention Trial (SELECT). JAMA 2011;306:1549–56.

15. Thompson IM, Goodman PJ, Tangen CM, et al. The influence of finasteride on the development of prostate cancer. N Engl J Med 2003;349:215–24.

16. Andriole GL, Bostwick DG, Brawley OW, et al. Effect of dutasteride on the risk of prostate cancer. N Engl J Med 2010;362:1192–202.

17. Pinsky PF, Black A, Grubb R, et al. Projecting prostate cancer mortality in the PCPT and REDUCE chemoprevention trials. Cancer 2013;119:593–601.

18. Wallner LP, DiBello JR, Li BH, et al. 5-alpha reductase inhibitors and the risk of prostate cancer mortality in men treated for benign prostatic hyperplasia. Mayo Clin Proc 2016;91(12):1717–26.

19. Catalona WJ, Smith DS, Ratliff TL, et al. Measurement of prostate-specific antigen in serum as a screening test for prostate cancer. N Engl J Med 1991;324:1156–61.

20. National Cancer Institute. Prostate-Specific Antigen (PSA) Test. Available at: https://www.cancer.gov/types/prostate/psa-fact-sheet. Accessed November 30, 2016.

21. Chybowski FM, Bergstralh EJ, Oesterling JE. The effect of digital rectal examination on the serum prostate specific antigen concentration: results of a randomized study. J Urol 1992;148:83–6.

22. Stenner J, Holthaus K, Mackenzie SH, et al. The effect of ejaculation on prostate-specific antigen in a prostate cancer-screening population. Urology 1998;51:455–9.

23. Mejak SL, Bayliss J, Hanks SD. Long distance bicycle riding causes prostate-specific antigen to increase in men aged 50 years and over. PLoS One 2013;8(2):e56030.

24. Greiman A, Shah J, Bhavsar R, et al. Six weeks of fluoroquinolone antibiotic therapy for patients with elevated serum prostate-specific antigen is not clinically beneficial: a randomized controlled clinical trial. Urology 2016;90:32–7.

25. Thompson IM, Ankerst DP, Chi C, et al. Operating characteristics of prostate-specific antigen in men with an initial PSA level of 3.0 ng/ml or lower. JAMA 2005;294:66–70.

26. Thompson IM, Pauler DK, Goodman PJ, et al. Prevalence of prostate cancer among men with a prostate-specific antigen level < or = 4.0 ng per milliliter. N Engl J Med 2004;350:2239–46.

27. Ankerst DP, Hoefler J, Bock S, et al. Prostate cancer prevention trial risk calculator 2.0 for the prediction of low- vs high-grade prostate cancer. Urology 2014; 83:1362–7.

28. Roobol MJ, van Vugt HA, Loeb S, et al. Prediction of prostate cancer risk: the role of prostate volume and digital rectal examination in the ERSPC risk calculators. Eur Urol 2012;61:577–83.

29. Catalona WJ, Partin AW, Slawin KM, et al. Use of the percentage of free prostate-specific antigen to enhance differentiation of prostate cancer from benign prostatic disease: a prospective multicenter clinical trial. JAMA 1998;279:1542–7.

30. Loeb S, Sanda MG, Broyles DL, et al. The prostate health index selectively identifies clinically significant prostate cancer. J Urol 2015;193:1163–9.

31. Loeb S, Lilja H, Vickers A. Beyond prostate-specific antigen: utilizing novel strategies to screen men for prostate cancer. Curr Opin Urol 2016;26:459–65.

32. Vickers AJ, Wolters T, Savage CJ, et al. Prostate-specific antigen velocity for early detection of prostate cancer: result from a large, representative, population-based cohort. Eur Urol 2009;56:753–60.

33. Vickers AJ, Till C, Tangen CM, et al. An empirical evaluation of guidelines on prostate-specific antigen velocity in prostate cancer detection. J Natl Cancer Inst 2011;103:462–9.

34. Vickers AJ, Thompson IM, Klein E, et al. A commentary on PSA velocity and doubling time for clinical decisions in prostate cancer. Urology 2014;83:592–6.

35. D'Amico AV, Chen MH, Roehl KA, et al. Preoperative PSA velocity and the risk of death from prostate cancer after radical prostatectomy. N Engl J Med 2004;351: 125–35.

36. Nickel JC, Gilling P, Tammela TL, et al. Comparison of dutasteride and finasteride for treating benign prostatic hyperplasia: the Enlarged Prostate International Comparator Study (EPICS). BJU Int 2011;108:388–94.

37. Andriole GL, Crawford ED, Grubb RL, et al. Prostate cancer screening in the randomized prostate, lung, colorectal, and ovarian cancer screening trial: mortality results after 13 years of follow-up. J Natl Cancer Inst 2012;104:125–32.

38. Shoag JE, Mittal S, Hu JC. Reevaluating PSA testing rates in the PLCO Trial. N Engl J Med 2016;374:1795–6.

39. Taylor KL, Luta G, Miller AB, et al. Long-term disease-specific functioning among prostate cancer survivors and noncancer controls in the prostate, lung, colorectal, and ovarian cancer screening trial. J Clin Oncol 2012;30:2768–75.

40. Schröder FH, Hugosson J, Roobol MJ, et al. Screening and prostate cancer mortality: results of the European Randomised Study of Screening for Prostate Cancer (ERSPC) at 13 years of follow-up. Lancet 2014;384:2027–35.

41. Schröder FH, Hugosson J, Carlsson S, et al. Screening for prostate cancer decreases the risk of developing metastatic disease: findings from the European Randomized Study of Screening for Prostate Cancer (ERSPC). Eur Urol 2012; 62:745–52.

42. Auvinen A, Moss SM, Tammela TL, et al. Absolute effect of prostate cancer screening: balance of benefits and harms by center within the European Randomized Study of Prostate Cancer Screening. Clin Cancer Res 2016;22:243–9.

43. Wolters T, Roobol MJ, Steyerberg EW, et al. The effect of study arm on prostate cancer treatment in the large screening trial ERSPC. Int J Cancer 2010;126: 2387–93.

44. Bokhorst LP, Venderbos LD, Schröder FH, et al. Do treatment differences between arms affect the main outcome of ERSPC Rotterdam? J Urol 2015;194: 336–42.

45. Essink-Bot ML, de Koning HJ, Nijs HG, et al. Short-term effects of population-based screening for prostate cancer on health-related quality of life. J Natl Cancer Inst 1998;90:925–31.

46. Heijnsdijk EA, Wever EM, Auvinen A, et al. Quality-of-life effects of prostate-specific antigen screening. N Engl J Med 2012;367:595–605.

47. Rosario DJ, Lane JA, Metcalfe C, et al. Short term outcomes of prostate biopsy in men tested for cancer by prostate specific antigen: prospective evaluation within ProtecT study. BMJ 2012;344:d7894.

48. Wade J, Rosario DJ, Macefield RC, et al. Psychological impact of prostate biopsy: physical symptoms, anxiety, and depression. J Clin Oncol 2013;31: 4235–41.

49. Loeb S, Carter HB, Berndt SI, et al. Complications after prostate biopsy: data from SEER-Medicare. J Urol 2011;186:1830–4.

50. Wilt TJ, Brawer MK, Jones KM, et al. Radical prostatectomy versus observation for localized prostate cancer. N Engl J Med 2012;367:203–313.

51. Hamdy FC, Donovan JL, Lane JA, et al. 10-year outcomes after monitoring, surgery, or radiotherapy for localized prostate cancer. N Engl J Med 2016;375: 1415–24.

52. Donovan JL, Hamdy FC, Lane JA, et al. Patient-reported outcomes in the ProtecT randomized trial of clinically localized prostate cancer treatments: study design, and baseline urinary, bowel and sexual function and quality of life. N Engl J Med 2016;375:1425–37.

53. Bokhorst LP, Bangma CH, van Leenders GJ, et al. Prostate-specific antigen-based prostate cancer screening: reduction of prostate cancer mortality after correction for nonattendance and contamination in the Rotterdam section of the European Randomized Study of Screening for Prostate Cancer. Eur Urol 2014; 65:329–36.

54. Gulati R, Gore JL, Etzioni R. Comparative effectiveness of alternative prostate-specific antigen–based prostate cancer screening strategies: model estimates of potential benefits and harms. Ann Intern Med 2013;158:145–53.

55. Roth JA, Gulati R, Gore JL, et al. Economic analysis of prostate-specific antigen screening and selective treatment strategies. JAMA Oncol 2016;2:890–8.

56. Wolf AM, Wender RC, Etzioni RB, et al. American Cancer Society guideline for the early detection of prostate cancer: update 2010. CA Cancer J Clin 2010;60: 70–98.

57. Smith RA, Andrews K, Brooks D, et al. Cancer screening in the United States, 2016: a review of current American Cancer Society guidelines and current issues in cancer screening. CA Cancer J Clin 2016;66:96–114.

58. Qaseem A, Barry MJ, Denberg TD, et al. Screening for prostate cancer: a guidance statement from the clinical guidelines committee of the American College of Physicians. Ann Intern Med 2013;158:761–9.

59. Basch E, Oliver TK, Vickers A, et al. Screening for prostate cancer with prostate-specific antigen testing: American Society of Clinical Oncology provisional clinical opinion. J Clin Oncol 2012;30:3020–5.

60. Carter HB, Albertsen PC, Barry MJ, et al. Early detection of prostate cancer: AUA guideline. J Urol 2013;190:419–26.

61. Moyer VA, U.S. Preventive Services Task Force. Screening for prostate cancer: U.S. Preventive Services Task Force recommendation statement. Ann Intern Med 2012;157:120–34.

62. Chou R, Croswell JM, Dana T, et al. Screening for prostate cancer: a review of the evidence for the U.S. Preventive Services Task Force. Ann Intern Med 2011;155:762–71.

63. Cho H, Klabunde CN, Yabroff KR, et al. Comorbidity-adjusted life expectancy: a new tool to inform recommendations for optimal screening strategies. Ann Intern Med 2013;159:667–76.

64. Crawford ED, Pinsky PF, Chia D, et al. Prostate specific antigen changes as related to the initial prostate specific antigen: data from the Prostate, Lung, Colorectal and Ovarian Cancer Screening Trial. J Urol 2006;175:1286–90.

65. Abdollah F, Sun M, Sammon JD, et al. Prevalence of nonrecommended screening for prostate cancer and breast cancer in the United States: a nationwide survey analysis. JAMA Oncol 2016;2:543–5.

66. Vickers AJ, Cronin AM, Björk T, et al. Prostate specific antigen concentration at age 60 and death or metastasis from prostate cancer: case-control study. BMJ 2010;341:c4521.

67. Schaeffer EM, Carter HB, Kettermann A, et al. Prostate specific antigen testing among the elderly–when to stop? J Urol 2009;181:1606–14.

68. Kim SP, Karnes RJ, Gross CP, et al. Contemporary national trends of prostate cancer screening among privately insured men in the United States. Urology 2016;97:111–7.

69. Catalona WJ, Hudson MA, Scardino P, et al. Selection of optimal prostate specific antigen cutoffs for early detection of prostate cancer: receiver operating characteristic curves. J Urol 1994;152:2037–42.

70. Powell IJ, Banerjee M, Novallo M, et al. Should the age specific prostate specific antigen cutoff for prostate biopsy be higher for black than for white men older than 50 years? J Urol 2000;163:146–8.

71. Rosario DJ, Lane JA, Metcalfe C, et al. Contribution of a single repeat PSA test to prostate cancer risk assessment: experience from the ProtecT study. Eur Urol 2008;53:777–84.

72. Salami SS, Vira MA, Turkbey B, et al. Multiparametric magnetic resonance imaging outperforms the prostate cancer prevention trial risk calculator in predicting clinically significant prostate cancer. Cancer 2014;120:2876–82.

73. Schoots IG, Roobol MJ, Nieboer D, et al. Magnetic resonance imaging-targeted biopsy may enhance the diagnostic accuracy of significant prostate cancer detection compared to standard transrectal ultrasound-guided biopsy: a systematic review and meta-analysis. Eur Urol 2015;68:438–50.

74. Klotz L, Vesprini D, Sethukavalan P, et al. Long-term follow-up of a large active surveillance cohort of patients with prostate cancer. J Clin Oncol 2015;33:272–7.

75. Tosoian JJ, Mamawala M, Epstein JI, et al. Intermediate and longer-term outcomes from a prospective active-surveillance program for favorable-risk prostate cancer. J Clin Oncol 2015;33:3379–85.

76. Overholser S, Nielson M, Torkko K, et al. Active surveillance is an appropriate management strategy for a proportion of men diagnosed with prostate cancer by prostate specific antigen testing. J Urol 2015;194:680–4.

77. Eggener SE, Badani K, Barocas DA, et al. Gleason 6 prostate cancer: translating biology into population health. J Urol 2015;194:626–34.

78. Ehdaie B. Active surveillance for prostate cancer: is it too active? BJU Int 2016; 118:343.

79. Weiner AB, Patel SG, Etzioni R, et al. National trends in the management of low and intermediate risk prostate cancer in the United States. J Urol 2015;193: 95–102.

80. Cooperberg MR, Carroll PR. Trends in management for patients with localized prostate cancer, 1990-2013. JAMA 2015;314:80–2.

81. Sepucha KR, Fowler FJ, Mulley AG. Policy support for patient-centered care: the need for measurable improvements in decision quality. Health Aff (Millwood) 2004;(Suppl Variation):VAR54–62. http://dx.doi.org/10.1377/hlthaff.var.54.

82. Han P, Kobrin S, Breen N, et al. National evidence on the use of shared decision making in prostate specific antigen screening. Ann Fam Med 2013;11:306–14.

83. Hoffman R, Couper M, Zikmund-Fisher B. Prostate cancer screening decisions: results from the National Survey of Medical Decisions (DECISIONS) Study. Arch Intern Med 2009;169:1611–8.

84. The SHARE Approach. Essential Steps of Shared Decision Making: Quick Reference Guide (Workshop Curriculum: Tool 1). 2014. AHRQ Pub. No. 14-0034-1-EF. Available at: www.ahrq.gov/shareddecisionmaking. Accessed April 3, 2017.

85. Six Steps to Shared Decision Making. Healthwise, INC, Web. Available at: http://cdn-www.informedmedicaldecisions.org/imdfdocs/SixStepsSDM_CARD.pdf. Accessed December 3, 2016.

86. Stacey D, Légaré F, Col NF, et al. Decision aids for people facing health treatment or screening decisions. Cochrane Database Syst Rev 2014;(1):CD001431.

87. Sepucha KR, Simmons LH, Barry MJ. Ten years, forty decision aids, and thousands of patient uses: shared decision making at Massachusetts General Hospital. Health Aff 2016;35:630–6.

88. Wexler RM, Gerstein BS, Brackett C, et al. Patient responses to decision aids in the United States. Intl J Pers Cent Med 2015;5:105–11.

89. Barry MJ, Wexler RM, Brackett CD, et al. Responses to a decision aid on prostate cancer screening in primary care practices. Am J Prev Med 2015;49:520–5.

90. Merenstein D. A piece of my mind. Winners and losers. JAMA 2004;291:15–6.

91. Barry MJ, Wescott PH, Reifler EJ. Reactions of potential jurors to a hypothetical malpractice suit alleging failure to perform a prostate-specific antigen test. J Law Med Ethics 2008;36:396–402.

92. McNaughton-Collins MF, Barry MJ. One man at a time–resolving the PSA controversy. N Engl J Med 2011;365:1951–3.

Screening Adults for Depression in Primary Care

Sarah Smithson, MD, MPH[a],*, Michael P. Pignone, MD, MPH[b]

KEYWORDS

- Depression screening • Depression treatment • Collaborative care
- Population health

KEY POINTS

- The burden of depression in the United States is substantial. A growing body of evidence supports the benefits of screening for depression in all adults, including older patients and pregnant and postpartum women, when coupled with appropriate resources for management of disease.
- Developing, implementing, and sustaining a high-fidelity screening process is an important first step for improving the care of patients with depression in primary care.
- Initial treatment for depression should include psychotherapy, pharmacotherapy, or a combination of both.
- Collaborative care models are evidence-based approaches to depression treatment and follow-up that can be feasibly initiated in the primary care setting.

INTRODUCTION
Depression: Epidemiology and Burden of Disease

Depressive disorders, including major depressive disorder (MDD), persistent depressive disorder, and other subsyndromal disorders, are important direct causes of morbidity and an indirect cause of mortality, in the United States and worldwide. The lifetime prevalence of depression has been estimated to be 10% to 15%. In the United States, 12-month prevalence for depressive disorders is 9.0%, and 3.4% for major depression.[1] Data from the National Health and Nutrition Examination Study (NHANES) collected from 2009 to 2012 suggest that 7.6% of the US population aged 12 and older had moderate or severe depressive symptoms.[2] Worldwide, approximately 350 million people are affected by depressive disorders, making it one of the top 3 causes of morbidity as measured by disability-adjusted life-years.[3]

Dr M. Pignone is a member of the US Preventive Services Task Force (USPSTF). The views expressed here are his and not necessarily those of the USPSTF.
[a] Department of Medicine, University of North Carolina–Chapel Hill, 102 Mason Farm Road #3100, Chapel Hill, NC 27514, USA; [b] Department of Medicine, Dell Medical School, University of Texas-Austin, 1912 Speedway Mail Code: D2000, Austin, TX 78712, USA
* Corresponding author.
E-mail address: Sarah_Smithson@med.unc.edu

Moderate and severe depression is associated with significant effects on quality of life, with impact in multiple domains, particularly social, work, and home functionality. Those with moderate or severe depressive symptoms were much more likely to report difficulties in these realms, compared with those with mild symptoms (74%–88% vs 46%).[2] Depressive disorders also have an enormous economic impact, estimated for the United States at more than $210 billion in 2010, up from $173 billion in 2005.[4]

Depressive disorders in adults begin to increase in prevalence in those ages 20 to 30, and continue to increase into middle age, with women more likely to be affected than men. In the United States, persons living below the poverty level are more than twice as likely to have moderate or severe depressive symptoms as those with higher incomes. After taking into account income, depressive symptom prevalence does not vary significantly across different races or ethnic groups. Depression is more common among those who are unmarried, divorced, or widowed, compared with those who are married; in those who have suffered traumatic life events; and in those with a family history of depression.[2] However, rates of depression remain significant even in those without these risk factors. Depression itself is associated with increased risk from other comorbid conditions, including cardiovascular disease.[5] Unfortunately, more than 70% of patients who screen positive for depression do not receive treatment.[6]

Who Should Be Screened?

The US Preventive Services Task Force (USPSTF) recommends screening all adults for depression.[7] The Task Force emphasizes that "screening should be implemented with adequate systems in place to ensure accurate diagnosis, effective treatment, and appropriate follow-up." The American Academy of Family Physicians makes a similar recommendation.[8] In contrast, the Canadian Task Force on Preventive Health Care (CTFPHC) does not recommend routine screening. The CTFPHC sites a lack of evidence on benefits and harms of screening in asymptomatic individuals, complicated by a concern for potential harms through false positives and unnecessary treatment.[9]

Special Populations

Older adults

For adults older than 65, the evidence base supporting screening is less robust due to a lack of trials specific to older adults. Nonetheless, in 2016, the USPSTF recommended screening in older adults based on the totality of the evidence across the age spectrum and called for more research into the best approach for screening and treatment in older adults.[7] Identifying depression in older adults can be more complicated than in younger adults, because depression may manifest as somatic complaints, such as weight loss, fatigue, insomnia, and poor concentration that mimic physical ailments common in older patients. Depression is also more likely to coexist with medical comorbidities, including cancer, neurologic impairment, arthritis, and cardiovascular disease.[10]

Pregnant and postpartum women

Both the USPSTF and the American College of Obstetrics and Gynecology (ACOG) note the particular importance of screening women during pregnancy and the postpartum period, when the risk of depression is increased.[7,11]

Screening Instruments

A variety of screening tests are used for depression screening in asymptomatic patients without a history of depression. The Patient Health Questionnaire (PHQ) is validated and widely used in a variety of clinical settings. The PHQ-2, a 2-question form of the PHQ, is popular for screening because it is brief and highly sensitive. An expanded form, the PHQ-9, also is commonly used (**Fig. 1**).[12]

Dozens of studies have examined the utility and diagnostic accuracy of the PHQ in clinical practice. A 2016 meta-analysis by Mitchell and colleagues[12] reviewed 40 studies and pooled data from 14,760 unique adult patients in primary care settings with a prevalence of MDD of 14.3%. Both the PHQ-2 (sensitivity 89.3%, specificity 75.9%) and the PHQ-9 (sensitivity 81.3%, specificity 85.3%) demonstrated good clinical utility as screening instruments for depression.[12]

Special Populations

Older adults

For older adults, a 2003 review of 18 studies in patients older than 65 compared 9 different screening instruments, including the Geriatric Depression Scale (GDS

PATIENT HEALTH QUESTIONNAIRE-9 (PHQ-9)

Over the last 2 wk, how often have you been bothered by any of the following problems?
(Use "✔" to indicate your answer)

	Not at all	Several days	More than half the days	Nearly every day
PHQ-2 1. Little interest or pleasure in doing things	0	1	2	3
2. Feeling down, depressed, or hopeless	0	1	2	3
3. Trouble falling or staying asleep, or sleeping too much	0	1	2	3
4. Feeling tired or having little energy	0	1	2	3
5. Poor appetite or overeating	0	1	2	3
6. Feeling bad about yourself — or that you are a failure or have let yourself or your family down	0	1	2	3
7. Trouble concentrating on things, such as reading the newspaper or watching television	0	1	2	3
8. Moving or speaking so slowly that other people could have noticed? Or the opposite — being so fidgety or restless that you have been moving around a lot more than usual	0	1	2	3
9. Thoughts that you would be better off dead or of hurting yourself in some way	0	1	2	3

FOR OFFICE CODING _0_ + _____ + _____ + _____

=Total Score: _____

If you checked off any problems, how difficult have these problems made it for you to do your work, take care of things at home, or get along with other people?

Not difficult at all	Somewhat difficult	Very difficult	Extremely difficult
☐	☐	☐	☐

Fig. 1. The PHQ-9. (*Developed by* Drs. Robert L. Spitzer, Janet B.W. Williams, Kurt Kroenke and colleagues, with an educational grant from Pfizer Inc.)

30-item and 15-item versions), the Center for Epidemiologic Studies Depression Scale, and the SelfCARE(D). These 3 common screeners all performed similarly with sensitivities of 74% to 100% and specificities of 53% to 98% for MDD.[13] The American Geriatrics Society recommends using a short initial screener, such as the PHQ-2 or GDS.[14]

Pregnant and postpartum women

The Edinburgh Postnatal Depression Scale (EPDS) includes questions about anxiety and excludes somatic symptoms, such as sleep disturbance, that are common after pregnancy, slightly increasing its sensitivity and specificity relative to the PHQ-9 in the pregnant and postpartum populations.[11] In its 2016 review, the USPSTF cited 2 US trials that supported an average sensitivity of the EPDS (≥13) of 0.80, yielding a positive predictive value of 47% to 64% in a population with 10% prevalence of MDD. They identified no studies of the accuracy of the PHQ9 in pregnant and postpartum women.[7] The ACOG advises use of "a validated screener," including either the PHQ-9 or the EPDS.[11]

Frequency of Screening

The optimal frequency of screening is not clear. Many practices repeat screening on an annual basis in those who have previously screened negative, but the effectiveness and efficiency of this interval (compared with others) has not been studied in trials. Patients with a recent history of depression should be monitored more frequently (see Treating Depression section, later in this article).

Benefits of Screening

A growing body of evidence supports the benefits of screening for depression when coupled with appropriate resources for management of disease. As early as 2002, the USPSTF published support for depression screening.[15] A meta-analysis of 7 trials, including more than 2400 patients, revealed that depression screening and feedback of the results to providers resulted in a 9% absolute reduction in the proportion of patients with persistent depression at 6 months compared with usual care. If the prevalence of treatment-responsive depression is 10% in primary care, then screening 110 patients would identify 11 depressed patients and yield 1 additional remission after 6 months of treatment. The signal for improvement was strongest when screening was coupled with adequate treatment and follow-up.[16]

An updated USPSTF recommendation in 2009 identified 2 new trials and emphasized that depressive symptoms are most improved when screening is coupled with changes in care delivery and treatment.[17] The smaller new trial (n = 59) provided only feedback on screening and found no improvement in depression outcomes.[18] A larger trial that included provider and staff education, expanded support staff roles, collaboration with behavioral health specialists, and follow-up contacts demonstrated a 10% absolute reduction in screen-positive depression at 6 months and a persistent 8% absolute reduction in depressed patients at 57 months.[19]

The 2016 USPSTF recommendation continued to support screening for depression. It recognized a general increase in resource availability among practices and removed any recommendations to limit screening to specific populations. It also recognized the need to support primary care providers and practices in modifying their care delivery to accommodate depression care.[7]

Harms of Screening and Treatment

Extensive literature reviews reveal little evidence on potential harms of screening for depression. Hypothesized harms, including treatment avoidance, deterioration in patient-provider relationship, labeling or stigma, and inappropriate or unnecessary treatment as a result of screening have not been borne out in any studies to date, although very few studies directly examined harms of depression screening.[20]

Harms of treatment initiated on the basis of screening are also important to consider. Psychotherapy and pharmacotherapy are both first-line treatment options.[21] Psychotherapy in various modalities (eg, cognitive behavioral therapy, problem-solving therapy) is generally safe and without major adverse effects other than the time required.

Pharmacotherapy is another option for initial therapy and is recommended to be included in regimens of patients who present with severe symptoms.[21] Rates of adverse effects vary by agent, and no agent is without potential adverse effects. Commonly reported adverse effects of second-generation antidepressants include gastrointestinal (GI) distress (6.4%–42.5%), headache (6.8%–38.3%), sleep disturbance (5.5%–31.0%), dizziness (3.9%–20.4%), sexual side effects (8.0%–73.0%), and weight gain.[22] More serious adverse effects include suicidal behavior (but not completed suicides), highest in younger patients in the month before and the month after starting treatment. Upper GI bleeding is another important potential adverse effect of selective serotonin reuptake inhibitors (SSRIs), with risk increasing with age. A 2014 meta-analysis that included 393,268 participants revealed an odds ratio (OR) of 1.66 (95% confidence interval [CI] 1.44–1.92) for GI bleeding in patients taking SSRIs. The risk of GI bleeding increased with concurrent SSRI and nonsteroidal anti-inflammatory drug use (OR 4.25; 95% CI 2.82–6.42).[23] In pregnant women, observational evidence supports that second-generation antidepressant use may be associated with a slightly increased risk of preeclampsia, postpartum hemorrhage, miscarriage, perinatal death, preterm birth, serotonin withdrawal syndrome, respiratory distress, pulmonary hypertension, congenital malformations, and infants small for gestational age. Cognitive behavioral therapy may be preferred by some women; its effectiveness has been demonstrated in multiple trials.[7]

IMPLEMENTATION OF THE SCREENING PROCESS

Developing, implementing, and sustaining a high-fidelity screening process is an important first step for improving the care of patients with depression in primary care. In this section, we examine some key aspects of the screening process.

Administering the Screening Instrument

As noted earlier, we recommend initial screening with the PHQ-2, based on its well-proven accuracy, short duration, and ease of administration. Practices have several options for how to administer the PHQ-2, including advance administration through a patient portal or written questionnaire that can be distributed to patients in advance of a scheduled visit, patient self-administration in the office in advance of the visit, nurse administration during check-in, or provider administration within the clinical visit. Each of these individual options has advantages and disadvantages (**Table 1**) and can be combined with one another in mixed approaches as well.

Patients who screen negative on the PHQ-2 and who have no history of, or current symptoms of, depression or related conditions require no further attention and can proceed to other aspects of their primary care visit. Those who screen positive should proceed on to complete the PHQ-9.

Table 1
Advantages and disadvantages of different modes of Patient Health Questionnaire (PHQ)-2 administration

Administration	Advantages	Disadvantages	Other Considerations
Advance self-administration via patient portal	High reach Low cost Ease of tracking results	Limited access to, and use of, portal Literacy concerns Concerns about administration of follow-up PHQ-9	Receipt and management of screening results Responsibility for follow-up
Advance self-administration via written questionnaire	Easier to implement Can be administered in waiting room	Literacy concerns Data entry burden on staff	
Nurse administration during check-in	Can be included in existing check-in process In-person administration can overcome literacy barriers	Fidelity with wording of questions can be challenging Competing nursing demands	
Provider administration during clinical encounter	Direct linkage to treatment decision-making In-person administration can overcome literacy barriers	Fidelity with wording of questions can be challenging Competing provider demands	

The PHQ-9 is designed for self-administration, and practices may choose to have their nurses or physicians ask their patients to self-complete the instrument during check-in or while waiting to see the provider. The nurse or provider should offer assistance to patients who may have difficulty completing the PHQ-9 due to limited literacy. Once completed, the nurse or provider should review and score the PHQ-9, recording the results in the health record (ideally in a discrete data field to allow for easier tracking). If necessary, the nurse should communicate the results to the provider.

Following up on an Abnormal Depression Screen

The PHQ-9 (see **Fig. 1**) has been shown to be helpful in identifying the severity of depressive symptoms (mild, moderate, or severe).[24] However, before treatment can be appropriately determined, additional assessment is warranted.

The *Diagnostic and Statistical Manual of Mental Disorders, Fifth Edition* (DSM-5) criteria for a major depressive episode require the presence of 5 or more symptoms to have occurred together over a 2-week period, that these symptoms "cause clinically significant distress or impairment," and that they are not better explained by another disorder (eg, substance misuse, a medical condition such as hyperthyroidism, schizoaffective disorder, or bipolar disorder).[25]

The PHQ-9 questions map well to the DSM-5 criteria, and the score provides an indication of severity, degree of functional impairment, and a useful measure to gauge improvement after treatment. Scores of 10 to 14 suggest mild symptoms, 15 to 19 moderate symptoms, and 20 or greater severe symptoms.[24] As such, the diagnostic assessment can begin with a review of the PHQ-9, followed by more specific questioning related to positive responses.

In patients with significant depressive symptoms based on the PHQ-9, it is helpful to check for symptoms of mania to differentiate bipolar disorder from unipolar depression. Mania is often characterized by symptoms like distractibility, irresponsibility or uninhibited behavior, grandiosity, unusual increase in activity (sometimes associated with weight loss), changes in libido, decreased sleep, and increased or pressured speech. If any of these symptoms are present, providers may wish to administer the well-validated Mood Disorder Questionnaire, a screening instrument specific for bipolar disorder.[26] Those patients with symptoms of mania should be evaluated by a psychiatrist, as should patients expressing delusions or other symptoms of a schizoaffective disorder.

Suicide is the most severe consequence of depressive disorders, and has been increasing in frequency over the past decade, with more than 42,000 deaths in the United States in 2014.[27] Assessment of suicidal thought is included in the PHQ-9 and providers and practices using the PHQ-9 should develop an approach for assessing suicidal risk for patients who report suicidal thoughts. Several potential risk assessment tools are available. In our practice, we have chosen to use the P4.[28] The P4 screener assesses "*past* suicide attempts, suicide *plan*, *probability* of completing suicide, and *preventive* factors" and stratifies patients into 3 risk categories: minimal, lower, and higher risk. The effectiveness of such an approach, however, remains to be demonstrated, a challenge made more difficult by the relative infrequency of completed suicide.

TREATING DEPRESSION

We have reviewed strategies for implementing screening and diagnosis of depression. Now we turn our attention to implementation of team-based treatment of depression through collaborative care, shown to improve treatment adherence, depression outcomes, and quality of life.[29]

Collaborative care models are evidence-based approaches to depression treatment and follow-up that can be feasibly initiated in the primary care setting.[30] Collaborative care is multidisciplinary, engaging both the primary care provider and another team member, usually a nurse, social worker, care manager, psychologist, or psychiatrist. The team uses strong communication methods via a shared electronic medical record, huddles, or team meetings to adhere to a structured management plan and close patient follow-up. In a variety of settings, collaborative care has been shown to be a cost-effective strategy to increase adherence, improve outcomes, and improve satisfaction of both patients and providers.[31]

Initial treatment

Initial treatment for depression should include psychotherapy, pharmacotherapy, or a combination of both.[21] It is important to partner with the patient to develop an individualized treatment strategy. Higher PHQ-9 scores reflect more severe symptoms, and patients with a higher symptom burden should be offered multimodal treatment initially. Patient safety always should be the highest priority, and indications of suicidality or psychosis should be explored and triaged to acute care settings or psychiatric consultation as indicated.

After assessing safety, take into account patient preferences and offer treatment. Pharmacotherapy is typically readily available. Medications can be prescribed by any licensed practitioner and there are multiple affordable first-line options. In the absence of specific preferences, treatment can begin with a low-cost SSRI.[21]

Patients and providers who choose psychotherapy should select a therapist based on local availability and the patient's financial resources. Multiple forms of psychotherapy have proven effective; patient choice appears important to the outcome. See forms of therapy in **Table 2**. Less intensive interventions, such as online cognitive behavioral therapy modules may be as effective as more intensive face-to-face options.[32]

When a patient successfully establishes care with a behavioral health specialist, following up on depression management remains a responsibility of the primary care team. Being a member of a robust "medical neighborhood" in which communication flows freely and effectively between primary care and specialists, including behavioral health providers, can improve access to behavioral health, facilitate a collaborative approach among providers, and create a support network for a particularly vulnerable population of chronically ill patients.[33] Informal relationship-building and formal contracts with local behavioral health specialists may improve patients' access to care and encourage consistent and timely communication between providers.

Table 2
Forms of psychotherapy

Form of Therapy	Brief Description	Intensity	OR (95% CI) of Remission
Face-to-face cognitive behavioral therapy (CBT)	Replace negative thinking with healthier thoughts	At least 6 sessions with therapist or psychologist	1.49 (0.90–2.46)
Face-to-face problem-solving therapy	Improve goal-oriented decision-making	At least 6 sessions with therapist, physician, or counselor	1.29 (0.83–2.02)
Face-to-face interpersonal psychotherapy	Emphasis on resolving interpersonal problems	At least 6 session with psychiatrist, psychologist, or nurse	1.37 (0.81–2.34)
Remote therapist-led CBT	Replace negative thinking with healthier thoughts	8–10 telephone or online sessions with psychologist or therapist	1.51 (0.98–2.32)
Remote therapist-led problem-solving therapy	Improve goal-oriented decision-making	6 telephone sessions with trained student or nurse	1.22 (0.23–6.57)
Guided self-help CBT	Replace negative thinking with healthier thoughts	3–4 self-guided sessions with minimal assistance from nurse or psychologist	1.73 (1.21–2.50)
No/minimal contact CBT	Replace negative thinking with healthier thoughts	Computerized	1.46 (0.96–2.23)

Abbreviations: CI, confidence interval; OR, odds ratio.

Data from Linde K, Sigterman K, Kriston L, et al. Effectiveness of psychological treatments for depressive disorders in primary care: systematic review and meta-analysis. Ann Fam Med 2015;13(1):56–68.

Follow-up of Treatment

During the acute phase of treatment, close follow-up can improve depression outcomes. Many organizations have developed treatment algorithms that include follow-up contact 1 to 2 weeks after the initial treatment visit (**Table 3**). This close follow-up is typically performed by nonphysician members of the care team, such as medical assistants, care managers, nurses, or social workers. The care team should follow-up on treatment in a stepwise approach, increasing the intensity of treatment every 8 to 10 weeks to achieve optimal depression outcomes.[30] After an inadequate response to initial pharmacotherapy, offer an increase in dosage, transition to an alternative agent, or recommend augmentation.[21] In our experience, stepped care is most successful when providers in the practice endorse the stepped care approach and have systems in place to support delivery of standard care.

INTEGRATING BEHAVIORAL HEALTH INTO PRIMARY CARE

Integrating behavioral health into the primary care setting removes significant barriers to providing comprehensive care for patients with depression. Traditional practices (least integrated) offer independent primary care and behavioral health services that rarely communicate with each other. Moderately integrated practices tend to be colocated but have not fully developed into a cohesive health care team. The most integrated practices are colocated and collaborate formally and informally to deliver care with a shared vision.[34]

Managing the Health of Populations

To achieve the highest level of effectiveness in screening and treatment of depression, practices and providers must develop systems to address care gaps outside of traditional office visits. Such systems require coordination of the roles of different team members, including development of standard care processes ("standard work"). It is essential to identify which care team members are responsible for non–visit-based population management and give them protected time to complete the work.

Several types of tools enable population health management of depression (and other chronic conditions). Some electronic health records allow a practice to identify patients diagnosed with depression and follow their symptom control over time. Discrete data entry of PHQ-9 scores allows a provider to trend an individual patient's response to treatment. On a population level, discrete PHQ-9 data entry allows the care team to identify patients with the greatest symptom burden. The creation of a depression registry (either paper or electronic) to identify and monitor these patients enables team members to proactively support patients rather than wait for patients to present to the office. Outreach efforts may include follow-up phone calls after visits to assess adherence to the treatment plan, identification of patients with poorly controlled symptoms for mobilization of additional care, including practice-based and community resources, and engagement of patients overdue for follow-up.

MEASURING IMPROVEMENT

Creating and sustaining a high-quality depression care program requires engagement in continuous improvement, including tracking of process, outcome, and balancing measures. Specific processes will vary from practice to practice, but there are basic measures that represent the foundation of solid depression management practices and can foster support for a collaborative care model, even in a fee-for-service environment in which team members' work is not directly reimbursed (**Table 4**). Practices new

Table 3
Acute phase treatment schedule with critical decision points (CDP)

CDP	PHQ-9 Baseline Severity Parameters	Treatment Modification	Treatment Options Designed for Medication Treatment Only. Psychotherapy for Mild to Moderate Depression Is Also Considered Evidenced Based
WEEK 0 *CDP 1*	Severity ≥10		Initiate antidepressant medication at lower end of the dose range.
WEEK 1 Phone call	If severity >20 or clinical concern		Evaluate patient status, initial response to therapy, medication tolerance; if PHQ-9 question 9 (suicide) was +, conduct Suicide Screening and assessment; May be from trained physician, therapist, nurse, or care manager. (If indicated, return appointment scheduled before week 4.)
WEEK 2 Phone call	Recommended for all patients (do PHQ-9)		Evaluate patient status, initial response to therapy, medication tolerance. Increase antidepressant dose to medium dose range, as tolerated. May be from trained physician, therapist, nurse, or care manager. (If indicated, return appointment scheduled before week 4.)
	PHQ-9 ≤5	None	
WEEK 4 *CDP 2*	PHQ-9 >5 and <10	Modify based on functionality and patient preference	Continue antidepressant in medium dose range, as tolerated. Communicate with psychotherapist about progress (if applicable). Consider switch to a different antidepressant if tolerability is an issue.
	PHQ-9 ≥10	Modify treatment	Schedule a return appointment for week 6. Consider switching to a different antidepressant. If no improvement at week 6, recommend switching antidepressant.
WEEK 6 Phone call	Recommended for all patients (do PHQ-9)		Evaluate patient status, response to therapy, medication tolerance. If PHQ-9 question 9 (suicide) was +, conduct Suicide Screening and assessment. May be from trained physician, therapist, nurse, or care manager. (If indicated, return appointment scheduled before week 8.)
	PHQ-9 ≤5	None	Enter continuation phase.

(continued on next page)

Table 3
(continued)

CDP	PHQ-9 Baseline Severity Parameters	Treatment Modification	Treatment Options Designed for Medication Treatment Only. Psychotherapy for Mild to Moderate Depression Is Also Considered Evidenced Based
WEEK 8 *CDP 3*	PHQ-9 >5 and <10	Modify based on functionality and patient preference	Increase antidepressant dose to higher dose range as tolerated. Communicate with psychotherapist about progress (if applicable). Consider switching to a different antidepressant.
	PHQ-9 ≥10	Modify treatment	Increase antidepressant dose to higher range if there has been a partial response. Consider switching antidepressant.
WEEK 10 Phone call	For patients who remain in the acute phase (do PHQ-9)		Evaluate patient status, response to therapy, medication tolerance. If PHQ-9 question 9 (suicide) was +, conduct Suicide Screening and assessment. May be from trained physician, therapist, nurse, or care manager. (If indicated, return appointment scheduled before week 12.)
	PHQ-9 ≤5	None	Enter continuation phase.
WEEK 12 (q 4 wk)	PHQ-9 >5 and <10	Modify based on functionality and patient preference	Increase antidepressant to higher dose range as tolerated. Communicate with psychotherapist about progress (if applicable). Consider psychiatric consultation.
CDP 4	PHQ-9 ≥10	Modify treatment	Increase antidepressant dose to highest dose. Switch antidepressant (if only had 1 antidepressant trial). Consider psychiatric consultation.[a]

Abbreviation: PHQ, Patient Health Questionnaire.

[a] Patients who do not achieve remission after 2 adequate 6-week to 8-week trials of antidepressants (shorter if unable to tolerate higher doses) should have a psychiatric consultation for diagnostic and management suggestions. Goal is 100% symptom reduction by week 12.

From Community Care of North Carolina. 2016 https://www.communitycarenc.org/media/related-downloads/ccnc-depression-toolkit.pdf ; with permission.

to collaborative care may start by focusing on a specific patient population, such as patients with diabetes or stroke, and then scale up their efforts over time. Work can be financially supported by billing for depression screening with Medicare G codes.[35]

Cost-Effectiveness of Screening

The cost-effectiveness of screening for depression remains controversial. Valenstein and colleagues[36] used a Markov decision analytical approach to model the

Table 4
Examples of process, outcome, and balancing measures in depression management

Measure	Description	Numerator	Denominator	Exclusion Criteria
Process measures				
Screening rate	% of all adult patients screened for depression	Adult patients completing depression screening tool in the last 12 mo	All adult patients managed by the practice	• Deceased • Diagnosis of depression
Appropriate treatment	% of adult patients with depression engaged in evidence-based treatment	Patients on an antidepressant or with a completed behavioral health visit	All adult patients with a diagnosis of depression managed by the clinic	• Deceased
Outcome measures				
Depression improvement	% of adult patients with depression whose PHQ-9 score has improved by 5 points or more since an elevated index PHQ-9 score	Patients with an elevated index PHQ-9 score whose subsequent PHQ-9 has decreased by 5 points or more	All adult patients with an elevated index PHQ-9	
Depression response	% of adult patients with depression whose PHQ-9 score has improved by 50% or more since an elevated index PHQ-9 score	Patients with an elevated index PHQ-9 score whose subsequent PHQ-9 has decreased by 50% or more	All adult patients with an elevated index PHQ-9	
Depression remission	% of adult patients with depression whose PHQ-9 score has decreased to <5 since an elevated index PHQ-9 score	Patients with an elevated index PHQ-9 score whose subsequent PHQ-9 has decreased to <5	All adult patients with an elevated index PHQ-9	
Balancing measures				
Clinical productivity metrics for team members	Productivity measures for team members engaged in outreach activities	Achieved clinical productivity units	Expected clinical productivity units	
No-show rate for depression follow-up visits	Rate of missed appointments for depression follow-up visits	No. of depression follow-up visits attended	No. of depression follow-up visits scheduled	

Abbreviation: PHQ, Patient Health Questionnaire.

cost-effectiveness of screening in primary care. They found one-time screening to have a cost-utility ratio of just more than $45,000 per quality-adjusted life-year gained. Periodic screening was not cost-effective compared with one-time screening. The results were dependent on the cost of screening, prevalence of depression, and rate and efficacy of treatment. Notably, this analysis did not assume implementation of the collaborative care model, nor did it account for reduced nondepression-related health care spending.

FUTURE CONSIDERATIONS/SUMMARY

Depression is a significant cause of morbidity and often goes without recognition or effective treatment. Screening has the potential to improve detection of depression. Coupled with a robust system for treatment that uses collaborative care, screening has the potential to reduce symptoms and improve quality of life and functional status. Despite evidence of effectiveness, depression screening remains incompletely implemented. Providers who wish to improve their effectiveness in implementation should implement a standard office approach to screening and diagnostic confirmation, followed by shared decision-making about treatment options. Providers also should develop a standard approach for follow-up to ensure treatment effectiveness (or implementation of an alternative approach if initial treatment is unsuccessful). The most effective approaches involve a multidisciplinary team, and use both in-practice and outside-of-practice care.

REFERENCES

1. Lépine JP, Briley M. The increasing burden of depression. Neuropsychiatr Dis Treat 2011;7(Suppl 1):3–7.
2. Pratt LA, Brody DJ. Depression in the U.S. household population, 2009–2012. NCHS data brief, no 172. Hyattsville (MD): National Center for Health Statistics; 2014.
3. Ferrari AJ, Charlson FJ, Norman RE, et al. Burden of depressive disorders by country, sex, age, and year: findings from the global burden of disease study 2010. PLoS Med 2013;10(11):e1001547.
4. Greenberg PE, Fournier AA, Sisitsky T, et al. The economic burden of adults with major depressive disorder in the United States (2005 and 2010). J Clin Psychiatry 2015;76(2):155–62.
5. Barth J, Schumacher M, Herrmann-Lingen C. Depression as a risk factor for mortality in patients with coronary heart disease: a meta-analysis. Psychosom Med 2004;66:802–13.
6. Olfson M, Blanco C, Marcus SC. Treatment of adult depression in the United States. JAMA Intern Med 2016;176(10):1482–91.
7. Siu AL, Bibbins-Domingo K, Grossman DC, et al. US Preventive Services Task Force (USPSTF). Screening for depression in adults: recommendation statement. JAMA 2016;315(4):380–7.
8. Maurer DM. Screening for depression. Am Fam Physician 2012;85(2):139–44.
9. Canadian Task Force on Preventive Health Care, Joffres M, Jaramillo A, Dickinson J, et al. Recommendations on screening for depression in adults. CMAJ 2013;185(9):775–82.
10. O'Connor EA, Whitlock EP, Gaynes B, et al. Screening for depression in adults and older adults in primary care: an updated systematic review. Evidence Synthesis No. 75. AHRQ Publication No. 10-05143-EF-1. Rockville (MD): Agency for Healthcare Research and Quality; 2009.

11. Committee on Obstetric Practice. The American College of Obstetricians and Gynecologists Committee Opinion No. 630. Screening for perinatal depression. Obstet Gynecol 2015;125:1268–71.

12. Mitchell A, Motahare Y, Gill J, et al. Case finding and screening clinical utility of the Patient Health Questionnaire (PHQ-9 and PHQ-2) for depression in primary care: a diagnostic meta-analysis of 40 studies. BJPsych Open 2016;2:127–38.

13. Watson LC, Pignone MP. Screening accuracy for late-life depression in primary care: a systematic review. J Fam Pract 2003;52(12):956–64.

14. Brown AF, Mangione CM, Saliba D, et al. California Healthcare Foundation/American Geriatrics Society panel on improving care for elders with diabetes. Guidelines for improving the care of the older person with diabetes mellitus. J Am Geriatr Soc 2003;51:265–80.

15. US Preventive Services Task Force. Screening for depression in adults: U.S. Preventive Services Task Force recommendation statement. Ann Intern Med 2009; 151(11):784–92.

16. Pignone MP, Gaynes BN, Rushton JL, et al. Screening for depression in adults: a summary of the evidence for the U.S. Preventive Services Task Force. Ann Intern Med 2002;136(10):765–76.

17. O'Connor EA, Whitlock EP, Beil TL, et al. Screening for depression in adult patients in primary care settings: a systematic evidence review. Ann Intern Med 2009;151:793–803.

18. Bergus GR, Hartz AJ, Noyes R, et al. The limited effect of screening for depressive symptoms with the PHQ-9 in rural family practices. J Rural Health 2005;21:303–9.

19. Wells K, Sherbourne C, Schoenbaum M, et al. Five-year impact of quality improvement for depression: results of a group-level randomized controlled trial. Arch Gen Psychiatry 2004;61:378–86.

20. O'Connor E, Rossom RC, Henninger M, et al. Screening for depression in adults: an updated systematic evidence review for the U.S. Preventive Services Task Force. Evidence Synthesis No. 128. AHRQ Publication No. 14-05208-EF-1. Rockville (MD): Agency for Healthcare Research and Quality; 2016.

21. American Psychiatric Association. Practice guideline for the treatment of patients with major depressive disorder. Arlington (VA): American Psychiatric Association; 2010. 10. Available at: http://psychiatryonline.org/pb/assets/raw/sitewide/practice_guidelines/guidelines/mdd.pdf. Accessed November 26, 2016.

22. Gartlehner G, Hansen RA, Reichenpfader U, et al. Drug class review: second-generation antidepressants: final update 5. 2011. PMID: 21595099.

23. Anglin R, Yuan Y, Moayyedi P, et al. Risk of upper gastrointestinal bleeding with selective serotonin reuptake inhibitors with or without concurrent nonsteroidal anti-inflammatory use: a systematic review and meta-analysis. Am J Gastroenterol 2014;109(6):811–9.

24. Löwe B, Kroenke K, Herzog W, et al. Measuring depression outcome with a brief self-report instrument: sensitivity to change of the Patient Health Questionnaire (PHQ-9). J Affect Disord 2004;81(1):61–6.

25. American Psychiatric Association. Diagnostic and statistical manual of mental disorders. 5th edition. Washington, DC: American Psychiatric Association; 2013.

26. Hirschfeld RM, Williams JB, Spitzer RL, et al. Development and validation of a screening instrument for bipolar spectrum disorder: the Mood Disorder Questionnaire. Am J Psychiatry 2000;157(11):1873–5.

27. Heron M. Deaths: leading causes for 2014. National vital statistics reports, vol. 65. Hyattsville (MD): National Center for Health Statistics; 2016. no 5.

28. Dube P, Kurt K, Bair MJ, et al. The P4 screener: evaluation of a brief measure for assessing potential suicide risk in 2 randomized effectiveness trials of primary care and oncology patients. Prim Care Companion J Clin Psychiatry 2010; 12(6). http://dx.doi.org/10.4088/PCC.10m00978blu.

29. Grochtdreis T, Brettschneider C, Wegener A, et al. Cost-effectiveness of collaborative care for the treatment of depressive disorders in primary care: a systematic review. PLoS One 2015;10(5):e0123078.

30. Unutzer J, Park M. Strategies to improve the management of depression in primary care [review]. Prim Care 2012;39(2):415–31.

31. Van den Broeck K, Remmen R, Vanmeerbeek M, et al. Collaborative care regarding major depressed patients: a review of guidelines and current practices. J Affect Disord 2016;200:189–203.

32. Linde K, Sigterman K, Kriston L, et al. Effectiveness of psychological treatments for depressive disorders in primary care: systematic review and meta-analysis. Ann Fam Med 2015;13:56–68.

33. Huang X, Rosenthal MB. Transforming specialty practice–the patient-centered medical neighborhood. N Engl J Med 2014;370:1376–9.

34. Heath B, Wise Romero P, Reynolds K. A standard framework for levels of integrated healthcare. Washington, DC: SAMHSA-HRSA Center for Integrated Health Solutions; 2013.

35. CMS. Decision memo for screening for depression in adults. Baltimore (MD): Centers for Medicare and Medicaid Services; 2011. Available at: https://www.cms.gov/medicare-coverage-database/details/nca-decision-memo.aspx?NCAId=251. Accessed November 30, 2016.

36. Valenstein M, Vijan S, Zeber JE, et al. The cost-utility of screening for depression in primary care. Ann Intern Med 2001;134(5):345–60.

Screening and Counseling for Unhealthy Alcohol Use in Primary Care Settings

Daniel E. Jonas, MD, MPH[a,b,*], James C. Garbutt, MD[c]

KEYWORDS

- Alcohol • Unhealthy alcohol use • Risky drinking • Alcohol use disorder • Screening
- Counseling • Implementation • Prevention

KEY POINTS

- Unhealthy alcohol use is common and is a leading cause of preventable deaths.
- Systematic reviews and evidence-based recommendations support screening for unhealthy alcohol use and subsequently providing appropriate interventions for people with risky drinking or alcohol use disorder (AUD).
- A single-question screen, the Alcohol Use Disorders Identification Test (AUDIT)–consumption (AUDIT-C), and the AUDIT seem to be the best tools for screening adults in primary care, considering accuracy and time burden.
- Behavioral counseling interventions delivered in primary care reduce unhealthy alcohol use for people with risky drinking behavior; more intensive interventions, including medications, are needed for people with AUD.
- Implementation of screening and appropriate interventions in primary care may require support systems, changes in staffing or roles, formal protocols, and additional provider and staff training.

INTRODUCTION

Unhealthy alcohol use is an overarching term that includes risky drinking and alcohol use disorder (AUD).[1–4] Risky drinking refers to consumption levels that exceed recommended limits and that increase the risk for health consequences.[5,6] The maximum recommended limits for adult men less than 65 years of age are 4 or fewer standard

---

Disclosure: The authors have nothing to disclose.
[a] Department of Medicine, University of North Carolina at Chapel Hill, 5034 Old Clinic Building, CB#7110, Chapel Hill, NC 27599, USA; [b] Program on Medical Practice and Prevention, Cecil G. Sheps Center for Health Services Research, University of North Carolina at Chapel Hill, 725 Martin Luther King Jr. Boulevard, CB#7295, Chapel Hill, NC 27599, USA; [c] Department of Psychiatry, UNC Bowles Center for Alcohol Studies, School of Medicine, University of North Carolina at Chapel Hill, CB# 7160, Chapel Hill, NC 27599-7160, USA
* Corresponding author. Cecil G. Sheps Center for Health Services Research, University of North Carolina at Chapel Hill, 725 Martin Luther King Jr. Boulevard, CB#7295, Chapel Hill, NC 27599.
E-mail address: daniel_jonas@med.unc.edu

Med Clin N Am 101 (2017) 823–837
http://dx.doi.org/10.1016/j.mcna.2017.03.011
0025-7125/17/© 2017 Elsevier Inc. All rights reserved.

drinks (**Fig. 1**) per day and 14 or fewer per week. The corresponding limits for adult women and anyone 65 years of age and older are 3 and 7, respectively. The fifth edition of the Diagnostic and Statistical Manual of Mental Disorders (DSM-5)[7] defines AUD as a single disorder based on meeting at least 2 of 11 criteria (**Box 1**). AUD can be characterized as mild, moderate, or severe. Unlike its predecessor, DSM-5 does not separate AUD into categories of alcohol abuse and alcohol dependence, and although those terms are used frequently in previous medical literature, they are no longer considered appropriate for use in clinical practice.

Unhealthy alcohol use is among the leading causes of preventable death in the United States, accounting for almost 90,000 deaths per year.[8–10] Only tobacco smoking and overweight/obesity result in more preventable deaths per year in the United States.[8] Epidemiologic literature has found that many health problems are associated with unhealthy alcohol use, such as cardiovascular problems (eg, stroke, heart disease, cardiomyopathy, hypertension), cancers (eg, gastrointestinal, head and neck, and breast), gastrointestinal problems (eg, cirrhosis, ulcers, pancreatitis), mental health problems (eg, depression, anxiety, suicide, cognitive impairment), neurologic problems (eg, peripheral neuropathy, cognitive impairment), fetal alcohol syndrome, motor vehicle accidents, and injuries and violence.[5,11,12]

With a prevalence greater than 20% among adults in the United States, unhealthy alcohol use is common.[13,14] However, drinking behavior varies significantly across states. For example, data from the Behavioral Risk Factor Surveillance System show that the prevalence of binge drinking over the past month (ie, men having 5 or more drinks on 1 occasion, women having 4 or more drinks on 1 occasion) ranges from less than 13.7% in 10 states (Utah, New Mexico, Oklahoma, Arkansas, Mississippi, Alabama, Tennessee, Kentucky, West Virginia, and North Carolina) to greater than 19.6% in 7 states (North Dakota, Nebraska, Iowa, Wisconsin, Illinois, Alaska, and Hawaii) (**Fig. 2**). Similarly, rates of abstinence vary by state: more than 54% of

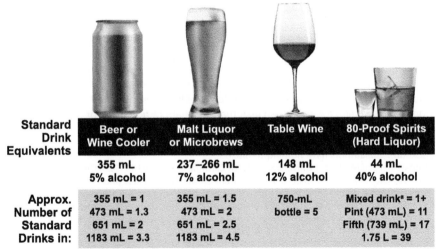

Standard Drink Equivalents	Beer or Wine Cooler	Malt Liquor or Microbrews	Table Wine	80-Proof Spirits (Hard Liquor)
	355 mL 5% alcohol	237–266 mL 7% alcohol	148 mL 12% alcohol	44 mL 40% alcohol
Approx. Number of Standard Drinks in:	355 mL = 1 473 mL = 1.3 651 mL = 2 1183 mL = 3.3	355 mL = 1.5 473 mL = 2 651 mL = 2.5 1183 mL = 4.5	750-mL bottle = 5	Mixed drink[a] = 1+ Pint (473 mL) = 11 Fifth (739 mL) = 17 1.75 L = 39

Fig. 1. What counts as a standard drink? [a] Note that, depending on factors such as type of spirits and recipe, 1 mixed drink can contain from 1 to 3 standard drinks. (*Data from* NIH. National Institute on Alcohol Abuse and Alcoholism. What is a standard drink? Available at: https://pubs.niaaa.nih.gov/publications/Practitioner/pocketguide/pocket_guide2.htm. Accessed March 1, 2017.)

Box 1
Diagnostic and Statistical Manual of Mental Disorders, Fifth Revision, diagnostic criteria for alcohol use disorder

1. Alcohol is taken in larger amounts or over a longer period than intended.

2. Persistent desire or unsuccessful efforts to cut down or control alcohol use.

3. A great deal of time is spent in activities necessary to obtain alcohol, use alcohol, or recover from its effects.

4. Craving, or a strong desire or urge to use alcohol.

5. Recurrent alcohol use resulting in a failure to fulfill major role obligations at work, school, or home.

6. Continued alcohol use despite having persistent or recurrent social or interpersonal problems caused or exacerbated by the effects of alcohol.

7. Important social, occupational, or recreational activities are given up or reduced because of alcohol use.

8. Recurrent alcohol use in situations in which it is physically hazardous.

9. Alcohol use is continued despite knowledge of having a persistent or recurrent physical or psychological problem that is likely to have been caused or exacerbated by alcohol.

10. Tolerance, as defined by either of the following:
    a. A need for markedly increased amounts of alcohol to achieve intoxication or desired effect.
    b. A markedly diminished effect with continued use of the same amount of alcohol.

11. Withdrawal, as manifested by either of the following:
    a. The characteristic withdrawal syndrome for alcohol.
    b. Alcohol (or a closely related substance, such as a benzodiazepine) is taken to relieve or avoid withdrawal symptoms.

Severity: mild, 2–3 criteria; moderate, 4–5 criteria; severe, ≥6 criteria.
Unlike DSM-III and DSM-IV, DSM-5 (American Psychiatric Association, 2013) describes a single alcohol use disorder category measured on a continuum from mild to severe, and no longer has separate categories for alcohol abuse and dependence. Diagnosis of alcohol use disorder requires at least 2 of the 11 criteria listed.
Data from American Psychiatric Association. Diagnostic and statistical manual of mental disorders. 5th edition. Arlington (VA): American Psychiatric Publishing; 2013.

---

adults drank no alcohol over the past month in 10 states, whereas roughly 40% or fewer adults drank no alcohol in 6 states (**Fig. 3**). In 2010, excessive alcohol consumption cost the United States an estimated $249 billion; about 75% of the cost was related to binge drinking.[15]

The United States Preventive Services Task Force (USPSTF) recommends that clinicians screen all adults for unhealthy alcohol use and provide persons engaged in risky drinking with brief behavioral counseling.[16] The National Institute on Alcohol Abuse and Alcoholism (NIAAA), US Department of Veterans Affairs, and American Society of Addiction Medicine (ASAM) also have recommendations for screening and providing appropriate interventions.[6,17–19] Despite all the evidence-based recommendations, most adults in the United States who visit general medical providers are not asked about alcohol use and most report never discussing alcohol use with a health professional.[20,21] Moreover, most patients with unhealthy alcohol use do not receive appropriate interventions. For example, data from the United States show that fewer than a third of people with AUD receive any treatment and fewer than 10% receive medications to prevent relapse or reduce alcohol consumption.[22–24]

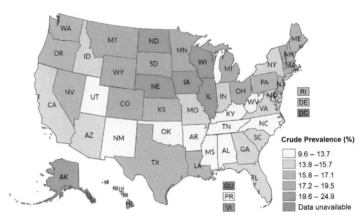

Fig. 2. Percentage of adults who reported binge drinking (men having 5 or more drinks on 1 occasion, women having 4 or more drinks on 1 occasion). (*From* Centers for Disease Control and Prevention (CDC). Behavioral Risk Factor Surveillance System survey data. Atlanta (GA): US Department of Health and Human Services; Centers for Disease Control and Prevention; 2014. Available at: https://www.cdc.gov/brfss/brfssprevalence/. Accessed November 21, 2016; with permission.)

This article describes evidence-based approaches for screening, identifying whether patients have AUD or risky drinking without AUD, and providing appropriate interventions for people who drink too much.

EVIDENCE-BASED APPROACHES FOR SCREENING

Systematic reviews and recommendations have established that multiple screening questionnaires can accurately detect unhealthy alcohol use in adults.[2,5,16] The 10-question Alcohol Use Disorders Identification Test (AUDIT)[25] is the most widely studied questionnaire (**Table 1**). Among the available instruments, the AUDIT, the

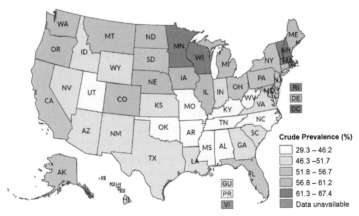

Fig. 3. Percentage of adults who had at least 1 drink of alcohol within the past 30 days. (*From* Centers for Disease Control and Prevention (CDC). Behavioral Risk Factor Surveillance Systemsurveydata. Atlanta (GA):USDepartmentofHealth andHumanServices; Centers for Disease Control and Prevention; 2014. Available at: https://www.cdc.gov/brfss/brfssprevalence/. Accessed November 21, 2016; with permission.)

Table 1
The Alcohol Use Disorders Identification Test

	Points per Response				
	0	1	2	3	4
(1) How often do you have a drink containing alcohol?	Never	Monthly	2–4 times a month	2–3 times a week	4 or more times a week
(2) How many drinks containing alcohol do you have on a typical day when you are drinking?	1 or 2	3 or 4	5 or 6	7–9	10 or more
(3) How often do you have 5 or more drinks on 1 occasion?	Never	Less than monthly	Monthly	Weekly	Daily or almost daily
(4) How often during the last year have you found that you were not able to stop drinking once you had started?	Never	Less than monthly	Monthly	Weekly	Daily or almost daily
(5) How often during the last year have you failed to do what was normally expected of you because of drinking?	Never	Less than monthly	Monthly	Weekly	Daily or almost daily
(6) How often during the last year have you needed a first drink in the morning to get yourself going after a heavy drinking session?	Never	Less than monthly	Monthly	Weekly	Daily or almost daily
(7) How often during the last year have you had a feeling of guilt or remorse after drinking?	Never	Less than monthly	Monthly	Weekly	Daily or almost daily
(8) How often during the last year have you been unable to remember what happened the night before because of your drinking?	Never	Less than monthly	Monthly	Weekly	Daily or almost daily
(9) Have you or someone else been injured because of your drinking?	No	—	Yes, but not in the last year	—	Yes, during the last year
(10) Has a relative, friend, doctor, or other health care worker been concerned about your drinking or suggested you cut down?	No	—	Yes, but not in the last year	—	Yes, during the last year
Total					

Data from Babor TF, Biddle-Higgins JC, Saunders JB, et al. AUDIT: the Alcohol Use Disorders Identification Test: guidelines for use in primary health care. Geneva (Switzerland): World Health Organization; 2001.

AUDIT-Consumption (AUDIT-C)[26] questions, and a single-question screen seem to be the best overall instruments for screening adults in primary care, considering accuracy and time burden.[2,5] Single-question screens and the AUDIT-C require just 1 to 2 minutes to administer. The 10-question AUDIT takes less than 5 minutes to complete. Some practices use a single-question screen or the AUDIT-C as a first step, followed by the 10-question AUDIT for those who screen positive as a second step (discussed later).

The NIAAA recommends asking whether individuals sometimes drink beer, wine, or other alcoholic beverages, and (if yes) following that up with a single question that asks how many times in the past year the patient has had 5 (for men <65 years old) or 4 (for women and those ≥65 years old) or more drinks in a day.[6] A response of 1 or more times constitutes a positive screen. For detecting unhealthy alcohol use, sensitivity of the single question is around 0.85 and specificity is 0.79, comparable with longer screening questionnaires.[2] Some health care systems or practices have published their experience with implementing and studying screening approaches that use the NIAAA-recommended question.[3,27]

The AUDIT-C is comprised of the first 3 items from the AUDIT and covers frequency of any alcohol use, usual amount, and frequency of heavy use. For the AUDIT-C, accuracy estimates vary by sex and cut point. For example, sensitivity is 0.86 and specificity estimates range from 0.72 to 0.89 for men when using a cut point of 4; sensitivity estimates range from 0.60 to 0.73 and specificity estimates from 0.91 to 0.96 for women when using a cut point of 3 (which are the cut points used by the Department of Veterans' Affairs for men and women, respectively).[2] The US Veterans Health Administration has implemented an evidence-based alcohol screening program that uses the AUDIT-C.[28,29]

In addition, the CAGE (cut-down, annoyed, guilty, eye-opener) questionnaire is well known to many providers because it has been available for more than 3 decades.[30] Although it is a reasonable tool for identifying AUD, it is not a good screening tool for the full spectrum of unhealthy alcohol use because it has low sensitivity for detecting risky drinking.[2]

SCREENING-RELATED ASSESSMENT

For patients with positive screening results, providers need to conduct screening-related assessments. The purpose of such assessments is mainly to confirm screening results and determine whether the patient has AUD versus risky drinking without AUD. In addition, screening-related assessments establish baseline behavior and may identify particular concerns to discuss when counseling. The assessment can be accomplished by conducting a diagnostic interview to ascertain whether the patient meets criteria for AUD (see **Box 1**). However, the time and training to conduct such an interview may be limited for primary care providers, and using certain support tools can facilitate screening-related assessment. For example, the 10-question AUDIT can be used as a next step for patients with a positive screen on the single-question screen or the AUDIT-C.[3,6,31] Then, the AUDIT score can be used to guide the assessment and subsequent plan. Total scores of 13 or greater for women and 15 or greater for men indicate a high likelihood of AUD.[3] In addition, for patients with total scores less than 13 (women) or less than 15 (men), a subscore of at least 2 points (total) from questions 4, 5, and 6 on the AUDIT indicates a high likelihood of AUD.[3] An alternative to using the AUDIT to guide screening-related assessment is a checklist provided in the NIAAA guide, "Helping Patients Who Drink Too Much."[6]

Screening-related assessment is essential for determining appropriate interventions. For patients with risky drinking who do not have AUD, counseling interventions in primary care are the preferred approach.[5,16] For patients with AUD, treatment options typically consist of referral to more intensive counseling programs (eg, 12-step programs such as Alcoholics Anonymous, motivational enhancement therapy, cognitive behavior therapy), detoxification, or pharmacotherapy. Counseling programs may use group counseling, individual counseling, inpatient or outpatient settings, and various other approaches.

COUNSELING FOR RISKY DRINKING IN PRIMARY CARE

Behavioral counseling interventions are designed to reduce or eliminate risky drinking. Effective counseling approaches include motivational interviewing, advice, feedback, alcohol consumption diaries, self-help materials, and problem-solving exercises to complete at home.[2,5] Systematic reviews have established the benefits of behavioral counseling in primary care after screening, showing significant reductions in alcohol consumption.[2,5] Compared with control groups, fewer adults who receive counseling report heavy drinking episodes (absolute difference of 12 percentage points) and more adults report drinking within recommended limits over 12 months (absolute difference of 11 percentage points).[5] The magnitude of improvement for health outcomes (as opposed to behavior change outcomes) is less certain because randomized clinical trials have not focused on health outcomes. Nevertheless, clinical trials have reported fewer hospital days and lower costs (benefit/cost ratio of 39:1 over 48 months; 95% confidence interval, 5.4–72.5),[32–34] and epidemiologic studies have consistently found both high average alcohol consumption and heavy per-occasion use to be associated with adverse health consequences.[5,12,35,36]

Brief (>5 minutes, up to 15 minutes), multicontact (≥2) interventions have the best evidence of effectiveness.[2,5] For such interventions, the number needed to treat (NNT) to get 1 person to change from risky drinking to drinking within recommended limits over 12 months is 7.[2,5] Project TrEAT (Trial for Early Alcohol Treatment) is an example of such an intervention.[37] It included a review of prevalence of risky drinking, feedback about health behaviors, information on the harms of alcohol, a worksheet on drinking cues, a drinking agreement or prescription, and drinking diary cards. The intervention was delivered in 2 visits with a primary care provider (15 minutes each). The visits were 1 month apart and each was followed up with a nurse phone call 2 weeks later.

Motivational interviewing techniques are often used in effective counseling interventions, and they are an effective patient-centered approach for achieving behavior change for a variety of conditions and settings.[38–40] Originally developed to address alcohol and other substance use, motivational interviewing uses a guiding style to facilitate behavior change by eliciting patients' motivations for change and by aiding exploration and resolution of ambivalence.[39,41] Reflective listening, open-ended questions, elicit-provide-elicit, asking permission, and importance and confidence exercises are all examples of motivational interviewing techniques.[3,39,41]

INTERVENTIONS FOR ALCOHOL USE DISORDER

For patients with AUD, several treatment options are available, and no single approach has been proved superior to others. Various treatment approaches have been reported to successfully achieve 1 year of sobriety for between 15% and 35% of patients.[42] Reported longer-term benefits at 3 to 5 years have been similar.[43] Twelve-step programs (eg, Alcoholics Anonymous), cognitive behavior therapy, motivational enhancement therapy, and pharmacotherapy are among the commonly offered treatments. At present, most of these are delivered in specialty settings, although colocation of primary care and behavioral/mental health services may be increasingly available in primary care settings. Most primary care providers traditionally have been trained to refer patients with AUD and have limited familiarity with counseling approaches and medications for AUD treatment.[44] Counseling for AUD may involve individual or group programs, inpatient or intensive outpatient programs, treatment centers, or other approaches.

Referral to 28-day residential treatment programs is an option for patients with AUD (typically those with moderate to severe AUD), but few trials have examined whether it is superior to outpatient treatment. One 3-arm randomized trial that enrolled 227 employees with AUD from an industrial plant found no difference for job-related outcomes (eg, being fired, job performance ratings by their supervisors) between those randomized to inpatient treatment, Alcoholics Anonymous, and a choice of options over 24 months of follow-up.[45] However, for measures of drinking (including continuous abstinence), the inpatient treatment was superior. Further, additional inpatient treatment was required more often (P<.0001) for those in the Alcoholics Anonymous (63%) and choice groups (38%) than in the inpatient treatment group (23%). Two other parallel but independent randomized trials conducted by the National Institutes of Health–sponsored PROJECT MATCH (Matching Alcoholism Treatments to Client Heterogeneity) compared cognitive behavioral coping skills therapy, motivational enhancement therapy, and 12-step facilitation therapy.[46] One trial enrolled subjects with AUD receiving outpatient therapy and the other enrolled those receiving aftercare therapy following inpatient or day hospital treatment. Both trials found that all 3 treatments improved drinking outcomes over 1 year, and found little difference in outcomes by treatment type. The trial of participants receiving aftercare reported higher rates of abstinence and longer survival to first drink than the trial of those receiving outpatient treatment.

Four medications have been approved by the US Food and Drug Administration (FDA) for treatment of AUD: disulfiram, acamprosate, oral naltrexone, and long-acting intramuscular naltrexone (**Table 2**).[1,47,48] The medications have not been studied for people with risky drinking who do not have AUD. The medications are generally recommended for maintenance of abstinence after a successful withdrawal from alcohol, in addition to psychological/counseling interventions.[49]

A systematic review that included numerous meta-analyses of pharmacotherapy for adults with AUD found that both oral naltrexone and acamprosate were effective for preventing return to any drinking (lapse) and reducing drinking days compared with placebo. Oral naltrexone was also effective for preventing return to heavy drinking (relapse) compared with placebo.[50] The NNT ranged from 12 to 20 for preventing lapse and relapse.[50] Meta-analysis of head-to-head trials that compared the two medications found no significant difference between them for lapse or relapse.[50] The most common adverse effects of acamprosate identified in meta-analyses of placebo-controlled trials included anxiety (number needed to harm [NNH], 7), diarrhea (NNH, 11), and vomiting (NNH, 42).[50] For oral naltrexone, they were dizziness (NNH, 16), nausea (NNH, 9), and vomiting (NNH, 24), respectively.[50] For naltrexone, the NNH for withdrawal from trials because of adverse events was 48; the risk was not significantly increased for acamprosate.[50] The effect sizes (NNTs and NNHs) reflect the added benefits of medications beyond those of psychosocial interventions and placebo, because the studies included in the systematic review included psychosocial cointerventions.[50] The medications have not been studied for use without such cointervention; future research is needed to determine whether medications are effective when taken without frequent behavioral interventions.[50] Future research on long-acting injectable naltrexone is also needed because the limited number of studies evaluating it leave some uncertainty about its benefits and harms. Nevertheless,

Table 2
US Food and Drug Administration–approved medications for alcohol use disorders

Medication	Mechanism	Dosing	Contraindications and Main Precautions
Acamprosate	Thought to modulate hyperactive glutamatergic NMDA receptors	666 mg (given as 2 333-mg tablets) 3 times per day	Dose reduction required for moderate renal impairment; contraindicated in patients with severe renal impairment
Disulfiram	Inhibits ALDH2, resulting in accumulation of acetaldehyde during alcohol consumption, which produces adverse effects such as nausea, dizziness, flushing, and changes in heart rate and blood pressure	250–500 mg once per day (often initiated at 500 mg and reduced after 2 wk)	Can cause medically dangerous symptoms with alcohol consumption
Naltrexone	Opioid antagonist: competitively binds to opioid receptors and blocks the effects of endogenous opioids such as β-endorphin	Oral: 50–100 mg once per day IM injection: 380 mg/mo	Contraindicated for patients with acute hepatitis or liver failure, and for patients using prescribed opioids or with anticipated need for opioids (can precipitate withdrawal and blocks effects of prescribed opioids)

The medications are typically prescribed for 3 to 12 months, but much longer courses are common in routine practice. Disulfiram was the only available medication from the 1950s until the 1990s, when oral naltrexone was approved.
Abbreviations: ALDH2, acetaldehyde dehydrogenase (the second enzyme in the alcohol metabolism pathway); IM, intramuscular; NMDA, N-methyl-D-aspartate.

long-acting naltrexone may be a good option when adherence is a concern or for patients who prefer a monthly injection instead of taking daily medications.

Many medications without FDA approval have been used or studied for treatment of AUD. The aforementioned systematic review evaluated 23 such medications, including antidepressants, mood stabilizers, anticonvulsants, alpha-adrenergic blockers, antipsychotics, and anxiolytics.[50] The review found some evidence supporting the effectiveness of nalmefene (an opioid antagonist similar to naltrexone that is approved in some countries for AUD) and topiramate. Compared with placebo, nalmefene reduced heavy drinking days (by about 2 per month, on average) and drinks per drinking day (by about 1, on average), and topiramate reduced heavy drinking days (by 9%), and drinks per drinking day (by about 1, on average).[50] The most common adverse effects of nalmefene identified in meta-analyses of placebo-controlled trials included dizziness (NNH, 7), headache (NNH, 26), insomnia (NNH, 10), nausea (NNH, 7), and vomiting (NNH, 17).[50] For topiramate, they were cognitive dysfunction (NNH, 12), paresthesias (NNH, 4), and taste abnormalities (NNH, 7), respectively.[50] For nalmefene, NNH for withdrawal from trials because of adverse events was 12; the risk was not significantly increased for topiramate.[50]

The medications are generally recommended for maintenance of abstinence, and most trials required patients to abstain for at least a few days before starting pharmacotherapy.[50] However, a few studies have reported reduction in heavy drinking for patients who were still drinking (rather than abstinent).[51–54] This finding is significant because some patients are not willing or able to abstain and some clinicians have advocated a harm reduction model, in which reduction of alcohol consumption (eg, reducing heavy drinking), improved physical health, or improvements in psychosocial functioning are considered viable treatment goals.[54–57] However, the harm reduction approach is controversial, and many clinicians think that abstinence is the only appropriate goal for patients with AUD.[56] Others have advocated for using a shared decision-making approach in which clinicians support patients as they clarify their preferences and values and discuss goals.[58] With such an approach, patients should be offered options for various evidence-based behavioral treatments, including medications.

IMPLEMENTATION OF SCREENING AND APPROPRIATE INTERVENTIONS IN PRIMARY CARE

Despite evidence-based recommendations, uptake of screening in many practices has been limited. Barriers to screening and providing appropriate interventions in primary care include lack of training and experience, competing priorities, misconceptions about the benefits of interventions, lack of confidence about being able to help patients with unhealthy alcohol use, and inadequate infrastructure. Health care systems or practices that have published their experience with implementing and studying screening highlight some of these important barriers.[3,27,28] Despite the barriers, some have successfully achieved high rates of screening.[3,28] For example, the US Veterans Health Administration has shown the ability to successfully screen more than 90% of outpatients using the AUDIT-C.[28,29]

Given that delivery of counseling interventions for people with risky drinking has been suboptimal, and that competing time demands in primary care are likely a key barrier, studies have evaluated whether counseling could be delivered by electronic interventions (e-interventions). A systematic review of 28 trials found that low-intensity e-interventions yield small reductions (approximately 1 drink per week) for adults and college students with risky drinking in alcohol use at 6 months, but found little evidence on longer-term outcomes or more clinically significant outcomes, such as meeting recommended drinking limits.[59] The included trials were not applicable to people with AUD and they were generally low-intensity interventions focused on giving brief feedback. Future research is needed to determine whether more intense e-interventions (ie, those structured similarly to brief, multicontact, in-person interventions) are effective for helping people reduce risky drinking.

Implementing systems for screening and delivering appropriate interventions for those who screen positive may require support systems, changes in staffing or roles, formal protocols, and additional provider and staff training.[3,5,28,50] The NIAAA has developed a clinician's guide called "Helping Patients Who Drink Too Much," along with related resources and training materials.[6] Some advocate using a chronic care management approach, similar to how primary care practices approach diabetes and other chronic diseases.[60] Given that interventions to reduce risky drinking and to treat AUD are significantly underused, providing them in primary care has the potential to reduce the substantial (and preventable) adverse health effects of unhealthy alcohol use. However, although studies of counseling for risky drinking after screening have shown benefits in primary care settings, clinical trials of AUD treatment in primary care, including those using pharmacotherapy, have reported negative or conflicting results.[50,61–66] Nevertheless, such studies have shown approaches to managing AUD in primary care that involve dedicated staffing and structure, and documented protocols.[50] Such studies used multidisciplinary team-based care, variations of chronic care management, and care coordination between primary care and mental health providers.[50] Some clinical trials conducted in non–primary care settings developed interventions with the intention that they could be used in or adapted for use in primary care.[50] The Combined Pharmacotherapies and Behavioral Interventions (COMBINE) Study's medical management intervention is one such example.[67,68] It consisted of 9 manual-guided counseling visits (45 minutes for the first and 20 minutes for the others) over 16 weeks. It is uncertain whether primary care practices could adapt to deliver counseling interventions requiring that much time; adjusting visit lengths or integrating behavioral health providers in team-based care may be required to do so.

SUMMARY

Unhealthy alcohol use is one of the top causes of preventable death in the United States. Given the preventable burden of disease and availability of well-validated screening instruments and effective interventions, reducing unhealthy alcohol use should be a high priority for health care systems and providers.

REFERENCES

1. Jonas DE, Amick HR, Feltner C, et al. Pharmacotherapy for adults with alcohol-use disorders in outpatient settings. Comparative effectiveness reviews, no. 134. Rockville (MD): Agency for Healthcare Research and Quality; 2014.
2. Jonas DE, Garbutt JC, Brown JM, et al. Screening, behavioral counseling, and referral in primary care to reduce alcohol misuse. comparative effectiveness review no. 64 (Prepared by the RTI International–University of North Carolina Evidence-based Practice Center under Contract No. 290 2007 10056 I.) AHRQ Publication No. 12-EHC055-EF. Rockville (MD): Agency for Healthcare Research and Quality; 2012.
3. Jonas DE, Miller T, Ratner S, et al. Implementation and quality improvement of a screening and counseling program for unhealthy alcohol use in an academic general internal medicine practice. J Healthc Qual 2017;39(1):15–27.
4. Saitz R. Clinical practice. Unhealthy alcohol use. N Engl J Med 2005;352(6): 596–607.
5. Jonas DE, Garbutt JC, Amick HR, et al. Behavioral counseling after screening for alcohol misuse in primary care: a systematic review and meta-analysis for the U.S. Preventive Services Task Force. Ann Intern Med 2012;157(9):645–54.
6. National Institute on Alcohol Abuse and Alcoholism. Helping patients who drink too much: a clinician's guide. Updated 2005 ed. Available at: http://pubs.niaaa.nih.gov/publications/Practitioner/CliniciansGuide2005/guide.pdf. Accessed March 4, 2015.
7. American Psychiatric Association. Diagnostic and statistical manual of mental disorders. 5th edition. Arlington (VA): American Psychiatric Publishing; 2013.
8. Mokdad AH, Marks JS, Stroup DF, et al. Actual causes of death in the United States, 2000. JAMA 2004;291(10):1238–45.
9. Centers for Disease Control and Prevention. FastStats: alcohol use. 2013. Available at: http://www.cdc.gov/nchs/fastats/alcohol.htm. Accessed December 5, 2016.

10. Stahre M, Roeber J, Kanny D, et al. Contribution of excessive alcohol consumption to deaths and years of potential life lost in the United States. Prev Chronic Dis 2014;11:E109.
11. Corrao G, Bagnardi V, Zambon A, et al. A meta-analysis of alcohol consumption and the risk of 15 diseases. Prev Med 2004;38(5):613–9.
12. Rehm J, Baliunas D, Borges GL, et al. The relation between different dimensions of alcohol consumption and burden of disease: an overview. Addiction 2010; 105(5):817–43.
13. Chen CM, Yi H-Y, Falk DE, et al. Alcohol use and alcohol use disorders in the United States: main findings from the 2001-2002 national epidemiological survey on alcohol and related conditions (NESARC). U.S. Alcohol Epidemiological Data Reference Manual, NIH Publication 05-57-37. Bethesda (MD): National Institutes of Health; National Institute on Alcohol Abuse and Alcoholism; 2006.
14. Vinson DC, Manning BK, Galliher JM, et al. Alcohol and sleep problems in primary care patients: a report from the AAFP National Research Network. Ann Fam Med 2010;8(6):484–92.
15. Sacks JJ, Gonzales KR, Bouchery EE, et al. 2010 national and state costs of excessive alcohol consumption. Am J Prev Med 2015;49(5):e73–9.
16. Moyer VA. Preventive Services Task Force. Screening and behavioral counseling interventions in primary care to reduce alcohol misuse: U.S. Preventive Services Task Force recommendation statement. Ann Intern Med 2013;159(3):210–8.
17. American Society of Addiction Medicine. Public policy statement on screening for addiction in primary care setting. 2005. Available at: http://www.asam.org/docs/default-source/public-policy-statements/1screening-for-addiction-rev-10-97.pdf?sfvrsn=0. Accessed November 30, 2016.
18. Management of Substance Use Disorders Work Group. VA/DoD clinical practice guideline for the management of substance use disorders. Washington (DC): Department of Veterans Affairs; Department of Defense; 2015.
19. Willenbring ML, Massey SH, Gardner MB. Helping patients who drink too much: an evidence-based guide for primary care clinicians. Am Fam Physician 2009; 80(1):44–50.
20. D'Amico EJ, Paddock SM, Burnam A, et al. Identification of and guidance for problem drinking by general medical providers: results from a national survey. Med Care 2005;43(3):229–36.
21. McKnight-Eily LR, Liu Y, Brewer RD, et al. Vital signs: communication between health professionals and their patients about alcohol use — 44 States and the District of Columbia, 2011. MMWR Morb Mortal Wkly Rep 2014;63(01):16–22.
22. Harris AH, Kivlahan DR, Bowe T, et al. Pharmacotherapy of alcohol use disorders in the Veterans Health Administration. Psychiatr Serv 2010;61(4):392–8.
23. Harris AH, Oliva E, Bowe T, et al. Pharmacotherapy of alcohol use disorders by the Veterans Health Administration: patterns of receipt and persistence. Psychiatr Serv 2012;63(7):679–85.
24. Hasin DS, Stinson FS, Ogburn E, et al. Prevalence, correlates, disability, and co-morbidity of DSM-IV alcohol abuse and dependence in the United States: results from the National Epidemiologic Survey on Alcohol and Related Conditions. Arch Gen Psychiatry 2007;64(7):830–42.
25. Babor TF, Biddle-Higgins JC, Saunders JB, et al. Audit: the Alcohol Use Disorders Identification Test: guidelines for use in primary health care. Geneva (Switzerland): World Health Organization; 2001.
26. Bush K, Kivlahan DR, McDonell MB, et al, for the Ambulatory Care Quality Improvement Project (ACQUIP). The AUDIT alcohol consumption questions

(AUDIT-C): an effective brief screening test for problem drinking. Alcohol Use Disorders Identification Test. Arch Intern Med 1998;158(16):1789–95.

27. Mertens JR, Chi FW, Weisner CM, et al. Physician versus non-physician delivery of alcohol screening, brief intervention and referral to treatment in adult primary care: the ADVISe cluster randomized controlled implementation trial. Addict Sci Clin Pract 2015;10:26.

28. Bradley KA, Williams EC, Achtmeyer CE, et al. Implementation of evidence-based alcohol screening in the Veterans Health Administration. Am J Manag Care 2006;12(10):597–606.

29. US Department of Veterans Affairs. Initiative QQER. Alcohol use screening clinical reminder. 2008. Available at: http://www.queri.research.va.gov/tools/alcohol-misuse/alcohol-clinical-reminder-screening.cfm. Accessed November 30, 2016.

30. Ewing JA. Detecting alcoholism. The CAGE questionnaire. JAMA 1984;252(14): 1905–7.

31. Jonas DE, Garza D. An evidence-based approach to screening and providing appropriate interventions for unhealthy alcohol use in primary care settings. J Comp Eff Res 2016;5(6):521–4.

32. Fleming MF, Mundt MP, French MT, et al. Benefit-cost analysis of brief physician advice with problem drinkers in primary care settings. Med Care 2000;38(1): 7–18.

33. Fleming MF, Mundt MP, French MT, et al. Brief physician advice for problem drinkers: long-term efficacy and benefit-cost analysis. Alcohol Clin Exp Res 2002;26(1):36–43.

34. Ockene JK, Reed GW, Reiff-Hekking S. Brief patient-centered clinician-delivered counseling for high-risk drinking: 4-year results. Ann Behav Med 2009;37(3): 335–42.

35. Bondy SJ, Rehm J, Ashley MJ, et al. Low-risk drinking guidelines: the scientific evidence. Can J Public Health 1999;90(4):264–70.

36. Shalala D, US Department of Health and Human Services. 10th Special report to the U.S. Congress on alcohol and health: highlights from current research. 2000. Available at: http://pubs.niaaa.nih.gov/publications/10report/intro.pdf. Accessed March 4, 2015.

37. Fleming MF, Barry KL, Manwell LB, et al. Brief physician advice for problem alcohol drinkers. A randomized controlled trial in community-based primary care practices. JAMA 1997;277(13):1039–45.

38. Lundahl B, Moleni T, Burke BL, et al. Motivational interviewing in medical care settings: a systematic review and meta-analysis of randomized controlled trials. Patient Educ Couns 2013;93(2):157–68.

39. Rollnick S, Butler CC, Kinnersley P, et al. Motivational interviewing. BMJ 2010; 340:c1900.

40. Rubak S, Sandbaek A, Lauritzen T, et al. Motivational interviewing: a systematic review and meta-analysis. Br J Gen Pract 2005;55(513):305–12.

41. Miller WR, Rollnick SR. Motivational interviewing: preparing people to change behavior. New York: Guilford Press; 1991.

42. Miller WR, Walters ST, Bennett ME. How effective is alcoholism treatment in the United States? J Stud Alcohol 2001;62(2):211–20.

43. Schuckit MA. Alcohol-use disorders. Lancet 2009;373(9662):492–501.

44. O'Malley SS, O'Connor PG. Medications for unhealthy alcohol use: across the spectrum. Alcohol Res Health 2011;33(4):300–12.

45. Walsh DC, Hingson RW, Merrigan DM, et al. A randomized trial of treatment options for alcohol-abusing workers. N Engl J Med 1991;325(11):775–82.

46. Project MATCH Research Group. Matching alcoholism treatments to client heterogeneity: treatment main effects and matching effects on drinking during treatment. J Stud Alcohol 1998;59(6):631–9.

47. Center for Substance Abuse Treatment. Incorporating alcohol pharmacotherapies into medical practice. Treatment improvement protocol (TIP) series 49. HHS Publication No. (SMA) 09–4380. Rockville (MD): Substance Abuse and Mental Health Services Administration; 2009.

48. Reilly MT, Lobo IA, McCracken LM, et al. Effects of acamprosate on neuronal receptors and ion channels expressed in *Xenopus* oocytes. Alcohol Clin Exp Res 2008;32(2):188–96.

49. The British Psychological Society and The Royal College of Psychiatrists. National Collaborating Centre for Mental Health, National Institute for Health and Care Excellence. Alcohol-use disorders: the NICE guidelines on diagnosis, assessment and management of harmful drinking and alcohol dependence 2011. Available at: https://www.nice.org.uk/guidance/cg115. Accessed December 5, 2016.

50. Jonas DE, Amick HR, Feltner C, et al. Pharmacotherapy for adults with alcohol use disorders in outpatient settings: a systematic review and meta-analysis. JAMA 2014;311(18):1889–900.

51. Garbutt JC, Kranzler HR, O'Malley SS, et al. Efficacy and tolerability of long-acting injectable naltrexone for alcohol dependence: a randomized controlled trial. JAMA 2005;293(13):1617–25.

52. Gual A, Lehert P. Acamprosate during and after acute alcohol withdrawal: a double-blind placebo-controlled study in Spain. Alcohol Alcohol 2001;36(5):413–8.

53. Kranzler HR, Armeli S, Tennen H, et al. Targeted naltrexone for early problem drinkers. J Clin Psychopharmacol 2003;23(3):294–304.

54. O'Brien CP, McLellan AT. Myths about the treatment of addiction. Lancet 1996;347(8996):237–40.

55. Caputo F, Domenicali M, Bernardi M. Medications for alcohol use disorders. JAMA 2014;312(13):1350–1.

56. Jonas DE, Feltner C, Garbutt JC. Medications for alcohol use disorders–reply. JAMA 2014;312(13):1351.

57. Keating GM. Nalmefene: a review of its use in the treatment of alcohol dependence. CNS Drugs 2013;27(9):761–72.

58. Bradley KA, Kivlahan DR. Bringing patient-centered care to patients with alcohol use disorders. JAMA 2014;311(18):1861–2.

59. Dedert EA, McDuffie JR, Stein R, et al. Electronic interventions for alcohol misuse and alcohol use disorders: a systematic review. Ann Intern Med 2015;163(3):205–14.

60. O'Connor PG. Managing substance dependence as a chronic disease: is the glass half full or half empty? JAMA 2013;310(11):1132–4.

61. Berger L, Fisher M, Brondino M, et al. Efficacy of acamprosate for alcohol dependence in a family medicine setting in the United States: a randomized, double-blind, placebo-controlled study. Alcohol Clin Exp Res 2013;37(4):668–74.

62. Karhuvaara S, Simojoki K, Virta A, et al. Targeted nalmefene with simple medical management in the treatment of heavy drinkers: a randomized double-blind placebo-controlled multicenter study. Alcohol Clin Exp Res 2007;31(7):1179–87.

63. Kiritze-Topor P, Huas D, Rosenzweig C, et al. A pragmatic trial of acamprosate in the treatment of alcohol dependence in primary care. Alcohol Alcohol 2004;39(6):520–7.

64. O'Malley SS, Rounsaville BJ, Farren C, et al. Initial and maintenance naltrexone treatment for alcohol dependence using primary care vs specialty care: a nested sequence of 3 randomized trials. Arch Intern Med 2003;163(14):1695–704.

65. Oslin DW, Lynch KG, Maisto SA, et al. A randomized clinical trial of alcohol care management delivered in Department of Veterans Affairs primary care clinics versus specialty addiction treatment. J Gen Intern Med 2014;29(1):162–8.

66. Saitz R, Cheng DM, Winter M, et al. Chronic care management for dependence on alcohol and other drugs: the AHEAD randomized trial. JAMA 2013;310(11): 1156–67.

67. Anton RF, O'Malley SS, Ciraulo DA, et al. Combined pharmacotherapies and behavioral interventions for alcohol dependence: the COMBINE study: a randomized controlled trial. JAMA 2006;295(17):2003–17.

68. Pettinati HM, Weiss RD, Miller WR, et al. Medical management treatment manual: a clinical research guide for medically trained clinicians providing pharmacotherapy as part of the treatment for alcohol dependence COMBINE monograph series. DHHS publication (NIH) 04–5289. Bethesda (MD): National Institute on Alcohol Abuse and Alcoholism; 2004.

Index

Note: Page numbers of article titles are in **boldface** type.

Med Clin N Am 101 (2017) 839–845
http://dx.doi.org/10.1016/S0025-7125(17)30076-7
0025-7125/17

medical.theclinics.com

Moving?

Make sure your subscription moves with you!

To notify us of your new address, find your **Clinics Account Number** (located on your mailing label above your name), and contact customer service at:

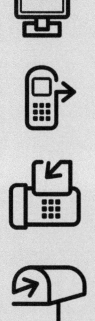

Email: journalscustomerservice-usa@elsevier.com

800-654-2452 (subscribers in the U.S. & Canada)
314-447-8871 (subscribers outside of the U.S. & Canada)

Fax number: 314-447-8029

Elsevier Health Sciences Division
Subscription Customer Service
3251 Riverport Lane
Maryland Heights, MO 63043

*To ensure uninterrupted delivery of your subscription, please notify us at least 4 weeks in advance of move.

Printed and bound by CPI Group (UK) Ltd, Croydon, CR0 4YY

03/10/2024

01040394-0017